The

Heart Smart

Healthy

Exchanges®

Cookbook

Most Perigee Books are available at special quantity discounts for bulk purchases for sales promotions, premiums, fund-raising or educational use. Special books, or book excerpts, can also be created to fit specific needs.

For details, write: Special Markets, The Berkley Publishing Group, 375 Hudson Street, New York, New York 10014.

The Heart Smart Healthy Exchanges® Cookbook

A HEALTHY EXCHANGES® COOKBOOK

JoAnna M. Lund

Introduction by
Susan M. Fitzgerald, R.N., M.S.

HELPing Others HELP Themselves
the **Healthy Exchanges**® Way™

A Perigee Book

A Perigee Book
Published by The Berkley Publishing Group
A member of Penguin Putnam Inc.
375 Hudson Street
New York, New York 10014

For more information about Healthy Exchanges products, contact:
Healthy Exchanges, Inc.
P.O. Box 124
DeWitt, Iowa 52742-0124
(319) 659-8234

First edition: February 1999

Published simultaneously in Canada.

The Penguin Putnam Inc. World Wide Web site address is
http://www.penguinputnam.com

Library of Congress Cataloging-in-Publication Data

Lund, Joanna M.
    The heart smart healthy exchanges cookbook / Joanna M. Lund ;
    introduction by Susan M. Fitzgerald. — 1st ed.
        p.   cm.
    "A Healthy Exchanges cookbook."
    Includes index.
    ISBN 0-399-52474-6
    1. Heart—Diseases—Diet therapy—Recipes.   2. Heart—Diseases—
    Prevention.   3. Food exchange lists.   4. Low-fat diet—Recipes.
    I. Title.
    RC684.D5L86   1999
    641.5'6311—dc21   98-33232
                                                          CIP

Printed in the United States of America

10   9   8   7   6   5   4   3   2   1

This cookbook, as all mine are, is dedicated in loving memory to my parents, Jerome and Agnes McAndrews, who both had hearts as big as the sky. While they never enjoyed the luxury of abundant monetary riches, they were wealthy beyond words in the love they shared with their family.

Our dinner table was always filled with both lively conversation and Mom's delicious fare. If we'd only known then what we know now, her family-pleasing dishes could have been heart-pleasing as well. And maybe Mom and Daddy could have enjoyed a few more years here on earth with their loved ones instead of both dying of congestive heart failure.

This book is also dedicated to everyone who must watch their diets because of cholesterol or heart concerns. The recipes in this book (all healthy versions of Mom's favorites) are heart healthy, but still family pleasing. Sometimes, when we discover that we must eat differently because of health reasons, we worry if we will be able to "do it." As usual, my mother had the perfect poem in her collection. May you enjoy both my mother's words and her daughter's recipes with your loved ones for years to come.

The Unknown Worry

Most people worry about the unknown things
that never take place,
Yet, we can't help seeing the anxiety
expressed on their face.
This is especially so when illness comes
and it is not clear
What is wrong or bothering a special friend
and those we love dear.
It is the unknown verdict we worry about
as we wait and pray,
But what a relief when the words finally come,
"Everything's O.K."

—Agnes Carrington McAndrews

Contents

Acknowledgments

Where do I begin, when my heart is so full of love and gratitude to so many for helping my dream of sharing "common folk" healthy recipes and a commonsense approach to healthy living with the world come true? I begin with:

God, for giving me the gift of creating recipes at a time when I needed them the most . . . when I started my own personal journey to good health.

Cliff Lund, for loving me for me and voluntarily choosing to become a part of Healthy Exchanges in both body and spirit.

Becky and John Taylor, James and Pam Dierickx, Tom and Angie Dierickx, and Zach and Josh Dierickx, for supporting their mother and grandmother in every way possible, from tasting recipes to washing dishes.

Marge and Cleland Lund, Mary Benischek, Regina Reyes, Loretta Rothbart, Juanita Dithmart, and Dale Lund, for being both loyal family and staunch supporters.

John Duff, for being the kind of editor that most authors only dream of working with.

Angela Miller and Coleen O'Shea, for helping me to realize that what I have to share with others is more than just recipes.

Barbara Alpert, for becoming a good friend as well as a top-notch writing partner.

Susan M. Fitzgerald, R.N., M.S., for seeing at once that my "common folk" healthy recipes are just what the doctor ordered.

Rose Hoenig, R.D., L.D., for making sure that the diabetic exchanges and the nutrient information is as accurate as it can possibly be.

Shirley Morrow, for faithfully typing and typing and typing and then retyping my recipes since the very beginning.

Lori Hansen, for calculating the nutritional values of each recipe and willingly doing it again and again when ingredients change midstream.

Rita Ahlers, for helping me test every recipe and keeping a smile on her face the whole time.

Everyone who has embraced Healthy Exchanges recipes and made them part of their family fare.

Introduction

All of us grew up eating and loving Mom's favorite recipes, and we'd like to keep doing so. The only problem is that those soul-comforting recipes of yesterday can mean real trouble for your waistline and for your arteries. I'm happy to report that help is at hand, in JoAnna Lund's *Heart Smart Healthy Exchanges Cookbook.* These recipes, which JoAnna calls "common folk healthy," are just like the great-tasting dishes Mom used to make. These tasty foods will appeal to *everyone* at the dinner table, they're not complicated to prepare, and best of all, they fit into today's busy lifestyle.

I've found JoAnna Lund's Healthy Exchanges cookbooks and newspaper columns to be a great resource for my patients. She provides exactly what people with cardiac concerns are looking for: a commonsense way to avoid deprivation by adapting the foods they *like* to eat. Not everyone is ready or willing to change to a low-fat vegetarian diet or prepared to spend the time in the kitchen that it takes to cook complicated, low-fat gourmet dishes. There are many heart-healthy cookbooks on the market, and I've recommended some of them for good ideas and special occasions. But this cookbook—and every one of JoAnna's books—is practical for *everyday* cooking. Being "smart" about your heart means making modifications in your diet *every day.* With JoAnna, you get exactly what you're looking for to help manage or prevent heart disease. If your goal is a lifetime of good health (and isn't everyone's?), you're taking a giant step in that direction!

What Does It Mean to Be Smart about Your Heart?

There have been hundreds of studies researching the causes of heart disease, many of which recommend taking specific steps to reduce your risk. But most people put off making the lifestyle changes needed to avoid developing cardiac problems (as well as high blood pressure, cancer, and diabetes) until something drastic happens—like a heart attack or emergency bypass surgery.

It's hard to know what or whom to believe. We're bombarded with countless headlines and pronouncements about how to stay disease-free. One says eat lots of grapefruit; another suggests you snack on walnuts; a third recommends you drink a glass of wine daily or exercise strenuously. Though much of this advice is good, it's better to remain just a bit skeptical of "quick fixes." It's never a good idea to favor the findings of a single study or try to reduce your risk of disease by focusing on a single risk factor. To be smart about your heart, learn all you can about a variety of ways to sustain good health and increase your longevity. No one can do it for you, but you'll get lots of help.

Risk Factor Reduction

You can take one of two approaches to reducing your risk of heart disease. If you're *reactive,* you'll wait to "react" until you've already had your first heart attack or been told you must have bypass surgery. Or you could take a *proactive* approach—and start learning about your risk *right now!*

Do you think you're too young to worry about heart disease? You're not. Many of the patients I work with are in their forties, some even in their thirties. Most of them are shocked to learn that people in the prime of their lives can have heart disease, and many never dreamed they'd have to cope with a serious health problem at such an early age. The good news is, confronting a health crisis encourages them to make major lifestyle changes—changes that result in a better quality of life than they enjoyed before experiencing a heart attack!

Do you know your risk factor profile? It's a good idea to assess your risks, including those that increase your chances of developing heart disease and *cannot* be altered. Let's start with those:

Age: Are you a man over 45 or a woman over 55? If you are, your risk is higher.

Gender: Are you a man? Men have a higher risk of heart disease, but the bad news is, women are catching up.

Family history of heart disease or sudden death: Did anyone in your family have heart disease or die of a heart attack? If so, you're more likely to suffer the same fate.

But don't become discouraged if you've answered "yes" to one or more of these questions. They're just the beginning.

Let's tackle the conditions or habits that can increase a person's chances of developing heart disease. These can usually be changed or controlled. They include:

- Cigarette smoking

- High blood cholesterol

- High blood pressure

- Physical inactivity

- Obesity

- Diabetes

- Stress or other emotional factors

Each person has a unique profile of risk factors, some more important than others. The best way to start *reducing your risk of heart disease is to talk to your personal physician.* Ask about ways to improve your condition through a change in diet, lifestyle, or exercise. Learn what resources (like this cookbook) are available to help you make these important changes. An eating program that's smart for your heart is a great place for everyone to begin.

What Is a Heart Smart Diet?

The American Heart Association (AHA) published its "Dietary Guidelines for the Healthy Adult" in the fall of 1996. The main goal of the AHA guidelines was the prevention and control of heart and blood vessel disease. Unlike many nutrition studies published annually, the AHA guidelines provide sound, consistent advice on heart smart eating. They deviate very little from the AHA guidelines published in 1988, although they do reflect advances in nutrition research over the past eight years. I'd like to summarize the important points for you.

Fats

The American Heart Association guidelines recommend a diet in which 30 percent of calories come from fat. Fifteen percent of that fat allotment should be in the form of monounsaturated fat. Though these guidelines are very specific, we don't need to go overboard calculating fat percentages on every mouthful we consume. The general idea is that we ALL should use fat sparingly. Read labels and choose foods that have 30 percent or fewer calories from fat. The monounsaturated fats are the good ones. Studies have demonstrated that they can actually help the liver reduce blood cholesterol levels. Polyunsaturated, hydrogenated, and saturated fats are the bad ones and should be avoided as much as possible. You may not believe it, but the saturated fat in foods has a far greater effect on your blood cholesterol level than does the cholesterol in foods (more about this later).

In response to all the negative publicity surrounding saturated fats, many food manufacturers have switched from butter and beef fat to vegetable oils. But, to give the vegetable oil a firmer, more butterlike consistency, hydrogen is bubbled through it, producing a hydrogenated oil. Hydrogenated fats or "trans" fats, as they are sometimes called, are just as bad for your health as saturated fats.

Here's some down-to-earth advice on ways to reduce your intake of artery-clogging fat:

- **Use fat sparingly.** See the Guidelines that follow for specific suggestions.

- **Practice, practice, practice reading labels.** Determine the amount of fat and type of fat per serving (but watch your serving size!).

- **Always know what you are eating.** Don't throw caution to the wind—focus on fat when you're at a restaurant, at a party, eating desserts during a celebration, or using high-fat condiments!

- **Try new recipes that are already modified for you** (like the ones in this Heart Smart cookbook).

- **Alter your own recipes by using less fat and choosing more unsaturated fat.** There are plenty of nonfat or low-fat substitutions on the market today. Use skim milk (instead of whole milk); nonfat sour cream, ricotta, or yogurt; egg whites (substitute two egg whites for one whole egg) or egg substitutes; applesauce or fruit purees in place of butter and oil in baked goods.

- **Alter the way you prepare foods** by trimming all visible fat; cooking with nonstick pans (to eliminate the need for butter or oil); chilling soups and gravies, then removing the congealed fat; and cooking with low-fat cheeses.

- **Alter your cooking methods** by grilling, roasting, microwaving, or poaching foods. Steam or sauté vegetables using water, broth, juice, or wine.

- **Purchase readily available nonfat versions of common foods** (dairy products, desserts, entrees). Watch the sugar content, though!

What about Cholesterol?

For years, people have been hearing that cholesterol is the enemy and that avoiding it at all costs is the best defense against heart disease. Today, we know that individual responses to dietary cholesterol vary widely, partly due to genetic differences and partly due to factors such as fiber intake, exercise habits, body weight, age, and menopausal status. Surprisingly, most of the cholesterol circulating in the bloodstream comes from the liver and not, as often thought, from the dinner plate. Despite the source of cholesterol (from the liver or from a cholesterol-rich meal), the body has several options to respond to it: (1) the intestines can absorb it, (2) the liver can turn down its own cholesterol production, or (3) the liver can convert some cholesterol to bile acids and other by-products ready for excretion. The degree to which these responses occur depends both on the cholesterol content of the meal and the genetic makeup of the person. But one thing is certain: The most important dietary culprit in raising blood serum cholesterol is saturated fat. Cutting back on saturated fat will have a greater impact on cholesterol levels than cutting back on eggs or cholesterol-rich foods.

Know Your Triglyceride Level!
Triglyceride levels in the blood are usually measured at the same time as cholesterol, but physicians rarely discuss them with patients. This is probably because it's believed that they cannot affect heart health on their own. However, it has become evident that high triglyceride levels do cause problems. High levels make the blood more viscous and sluggish; thus, less oxygen and fewer nutrients are sent to the heart muscle. Though a triglyceride concentration that falls below 200 is considered normal, some studies suggest that individuals with triglyceride levels greater than 100 have twice the risk of heart disease than those with lower levels.

The important thing to remember is that triglycerides are fats. These levels can vary greatly, depending on what was on the dinner table last night. Happily, they are more responsive to Heart Smart eating and lifestyle changes than your cholesterol levels. To reduce your triglyceride level, here are four things you can do: (1) follow a low-fat diet, (2) lose excess weight, (3) avoid alcohol, and (4) restrict simple carbohydrates. Excess simple carbohydrates (beyond your daily calorie needs) are turned into triglycerides in the liver. Sugar, honey, and syrups are commonly used simple carbohydrates, but beware of the hidden sugars in fat-free but still sugary desserts and snack items!

What's All This Talk about Antioxidants?
Vitamins C, E, and beta-carotene are called antioxidants. Antioxidants work to neutralize substances called free radicals that result from your cells' ordinary metabolism. Scientists think damage from free radicals may contribute to cardiovascular disease. However, studies haven't proven conclusively that antioxidant supplements protect against heart disease.

Of all the antioxidants, vitamin E shows the most promise for protection against heart disease. Vitamin E is a potent antioxidant that attaches directly to low-density lipoprotein (LDL), or "bad," cholesterol and helps prevent damage from free radicals. Studies show that 400 IU of vitamin E daily might prevent or slow the progression of atherosclerosis in people with heart disease. The flip side is that high doses of vitamin E can cause bleeding and other complications. Moreover, there are many forms of vitamin E on the market, so it's difficult to know which is the best choice. I recommend checking with your physician before taking a vitamin E supplement. Remember, any benefit antioxidants offer against heart disease is much less than you can get from following a Heart Smart diet and making time for regular exercise.

Increase Your Fiber Intake

Fiber is one of the newer "buzzwords" in the fight against heart disease. Getting more fiber in your diet is a good prescription for all of us. What does that mean? Eat plenty of fruits, vegetables, dried beans and legumes (such as black beans, lentils, split peas), and whole-grain products (whole-wheat bread, brown rice, whole-grain cereals). The soluble fiber found in these products can help reduce LDL cholesterol. Studies have demonstrated a decreased risk of heart disease, as well as cancer, in individuals who consume 25 to 30 grams of fiber a day from food, *not* supplements.

Avoid Foods High in Sugar

Beware of fat-free baked goods. They are usually high in sugar! Foods high in sugar have no nutritional value and provide empty calories. They may initially give you energy and decrease your hunger but will cause fatigue and sluggishness later on. Moreover, even as little as one fat-free cookie or coffee with sugar in it can diminish your appetite for healthful foods such as vegetables and whole grains; also, high-sugar foods may have harmful effects on your blood-fat levels. You'll feel better, more energetic, and healthier if you eat foods that are low in fat and sugar, and rich in complex carbohydrates and protein. Try to ensure that everything you eat has some nutritional value!

Avoid Foods High in Sodium

Many people have to monitor their sodium intake for medical reasons (high blood pressure, kidney problems, and heart disease). However, even if your physician has not asked you to restrict your sodium intake, moderation is your best bet. Like fat, the sodium content of many foods far exceeds our recommended intake. Aside from readily available labeled foods that must state how much sodium is in each serving, there are many high-sodium foods prepared and saturated in salt. Fast food, packaged rice and noodle mixes, and soups are good examples.

Try using herbs and spices to enhance the flavors in your cooking. Substitute low-sodium and salt-free choices that are available at most grocery stores. If you have chosen to eat a high-sodium product at one meal, regulate your intake the rest of the day to compensate for it. Awareness is the key. Know what you are preparing when you cook at home; know what you are ordering when you dine out, know what you are eating at each and every meal. Be conscientious, and use salt sparingly!

What Else Can You Do?

Eating sensibly is only part of the equation when your goal is preventing heart disease or recovering from a heart attack. There is more you can do to live a healthy life and feel good for a lifetime.

Maintain a healthy weight.
Being overweight is associated with a variety of health problems, including heart disease. Getting down to a healthy weight is essential to maintaining good health. Even a loss of 10 to 15 percent of your starting weight can produce a dramatic effect in most obese individuals with high blood pressure or diabetes. Sometimes, these patients can reduce or discontinue their antihypertensive medication.

Losing weight is always a challenge, but the difficult part is keeping the weight off. This can only be achieved by making lifestyle and behavioral changes (not by crash diets, which result in repeated losing and regaining of weight and can be even more dangerous to your health than overweight!). The key to successful weight loss is to maintain a balanced Heart Smart diet, shed excess pounds slowly, increase physical activity, and become aware of the cues that stimulate inappropriate eating.

Be active.

Our bodies were meant to move. If they weren't, we wouldn't be built as we are and would more likely look like turtles or hippos! Sedentary lifestyles go hand in hand with unhealthy diets and numerous cardiac risk factors.

Are you sedentary? Answer these questions:

- Do you exercise 20 to 30 minutes at least three times weekly?

- Do your leisure-time activities require you to move from place to place?

Did you answer no to either of those questions? Okay, try these:

- Do you spend most of your day sitting?

- Do you have a job that is inactive?

- Do you seldom walk more than one block each day?

Did you answer yes to any of those? If you answered no to the first two and yes to the others, you are considered sedentary—and you need to make some changes!

Increasing physical activity is a prime example of how a risk-reducing behavior can have multiple benefits. In addition to improving cardiovascular health, regular exercise promotes weight loss, helps lower blood pressure, and enhances the body's ability to eliminate cholesterol and other fatty substances. It even reduces the lifestyle-limiting effects of osteoporosis and arthritis, improves mental health, and helps us remain independent as we age, improving the quality of life. In other words, physical activity delays the onset of, and reduces the severity of, the natural consequences of aging.

The traditional exercise prescription for cardiovascular health is 20 to 40 minutes of moderate- to high-intensity aerobic activity (running, cycling, swimming) done 3 to 5 times weekly. Unfortunately, most people don't follow this prescription for optimum health to the letter.

The good news is that studies have also shown that the traditional definition of exercise as a "high performance" workout has changed in recent years. Now it's recommended that every adult accumulate 30 minutes or more of moderate-intensity physical activity (to include recreational walking or gardening) on most, preferably all, days of the week. These recommendations are based on evidence that *health benefits are gained from any increase in physical activity*. But these revised recommendations are meant to complement, not replace, the traditional exercise prescription. Moderate to vigorous exercise will provide even more health benefits in the long run.

Here are some principles to get you started:

- **Play around.** Choose a sport that you enjoy, and get back into it. Dance, bike, play in the water or snow, run with the dogs.

- **Find an interest.** Become an expert at something you've always been interested in. Take a hike, go to the museum or on a day trip, garden, take an active vacation, explore architecture or bird-watching.

- **Use diversion.** Exercise with a friend, take a fitness class, entertain yourself while you work out (use a Walkman, read a book, listen to a tape, or watch TV while using gym equipment, play mental games, solve problems, fantasize).

- **Spice it up.** Regularly vary your type of exercise, time of day, and route. Improvise by walking to a destination you usually ride to, or walking home after getting a ride there.

Reduce the stress in your life.
Cardiovascular health has an emotional component. If you're constantly under pressure, coping with anxiety, dealing with people or things that upset you, your body feels it. If it gets to be more than you can handle, your body suffers. And if you're already at risk for developing heart disease, you need to find ways to lower the impact of stress in your everyday life.

What can you do? Besides eating well and getting moderate exercise, you should:

- Make sure you're getting sufficient sleep. Sometimes a nap is just the thing!

- Find ways to relieve pressure by taking breaks at work (a short walk after meeting with a difficult client) or making time to relax at home (listening to music, taking a leisurely bath instead of a quick shower).

- Try to spend more time with the people who make you feel good about yourself and less time with those who make you angry or unhappy.

- Set aside time to reconnect with your religious faith, or if you prefer, meditate privately.

- Take mental vacations. Read a book just for fun, or rent a silly movie and watch it with your family gathered around.

- Ask for help. Everyone needs it sometimes, and going it alone can be more than exhausting—it can be dangerous to your health. Maybe it means delegating more at work, setting up a chore-sharing chart at home, or even consulting a counselor or clergyperson.

Living well for a lifetime—what could be better than that? You've taken an important first step by choosing this book to help you reduce your risk factors for heart disease, but don't stop there; do all you can to improve your overall health and longevity. It's up to you to make the changes—but I know you can do it. Start today—do it NOW!

—Susan M. Fitzgerald, R.N., M.S.

Guidelines for

Heart Smart Eating

These recommendations focus on providing guidelines for selecting lower-saturated-fat foods.

- Limit high-fat animal products and palm, coconut, hydrogenated and partially hydrogenated oils (these fats increase LDL or "bad" cholesterol).

- Focus on "good" fats—e.g., fish, olive, and canola oils; walnuts; almonds; pecans; pistachios; and filberts (these fats help increase or maintain HDL, or "good" cholesterol).

- Select a variety from each food group.

Lower Saturated Fat	Higher Saturated Fat
(Choose more often)	(Choose less often and in smaller amounts)
Breads, Cereals, and Grains	**Breads, Cereals, and Grains**
Breads and rolls: whole-wheat, white, rye, and pumpernickel breads; bagels; English muffins; sandwich buns; dinner rolls	*Bread and rolls*: croissants, butter rolls, sweet rolls, Danish pastry, doughnuts
Cereal: most hot and cold cereals that are low in fat and sugar	*Cereal*: granola cereals made with saturated fat
Noodles and rice: all varieties of plain noodles and rice	*Noodles and rice*: noodles, macaroni, spaghetti, or rice prepared in butter, cream, or cheese sauce

Lower Saturated Fat	Higher Saturated Fat

Fruits and Vegetables

All varieties of fresh, frozen, canned, or dried fruits and vegetables

Sweets and Snacks

Frozen desserts: varieties with 3 grams of fat or less per ½-cup serving

Cake: angel food and other varieties with 3 grams of fat or less per serving (a serving is one piece 2 by 2 by 2 inches thick)

Cookies: varieties with 2 grams of fat or less in 2 small or 1 large cookie (includes fruit bars, ginger snaps, and vanilla wafers)

Candy: hard candy, jelly beans, gumdrops, marshmallows

Snack foods*: crackers with 2 grams of fat or less per ½-ounce serving; plain or low-fat microwave popcorn, pretzels

Dairy Products and Eggs

Milk: skim or 1% milk, low-fat buttermilk, chocolate-flavored skim milk, evaporated skim milk

*high in sodium

Fruits and Vegetables

Vegetables prepared in butter, cream, or cheese sauce

Sweets and Snacks

Frozen desserts: ice cream and other frozen desserts with more than 3 grams of fat per ½ cup

Cakes or pies: frosted cakes, pound cake, most store-bought cakes and pies, cheesecake, and other varieties with more than 3 grams of fat per serving (a serving is one piece 2 by 2 by 2 inches thick)

Cookies: varieties with more than 2 grams of fat in 2 small or 1 large cookie

Candy: chocolate, candy bars, fudge

Snack foods*: crackers with more than 2 grams of fat per ½-ounce serving, most commercial snack foods (like potato or corn chips, cheese puffs, etc.), buttered or regular microwave popcorn

Dairy Products and Eggs

Milk: whole or 2% milk, condensed or evaporated whole milk, cream, half & half, whipped cream, sour cream, non-dairy creamer or topping

Lower Saturated Fat

Dairy Products and Eggs (continued)

Cheese*: low-fat cottage cheese, hard cheeses with 5 grams of fat or less per ounce
Yogurt: nonfat or 1% fat yogurt, plain or flavored
Eggs: egg yolks (4 egg yolks per week, 1 if your cholesterol level is elevated), egg whites

Fats and Oils

Vegetable oil: olive, canola
Margarine: brands made with unsaturated oils; first ingredient should be water
Salad dressing and mayonnaise: salad dressing and mayonnaise with 3 grams of fat or less per tablespoon
Nuts: walnuts, almonds, pecans, pistachios, filberts

Meats

Beef: (all visible fat removed) diet-lean (90% or leaner) or extra-lean ground beef, lean cuts like round, sirloin, chuck, or loin
Pork: (all fat removed) lean cuts like tenderloin, leg, shoulder (arm or picnic); ham*; Canadian bacon*

Higher Saturated Fat

Dairy Products and Eggs (continued)

Cheese*: regular cottage cheese, cream cheese, cheese spreads, hard cheeses with more than 5 grams of fat per ounce
Yogurt: yogurt made from whole or 2% milk

Fats and Oils

Fats and oils: solid vegetable shortening, hydrogenated and partially hydrogenated oils, lard, bacon fat, coconut and palm oils; unsaturated oils like corn, peanut, safflower, sesame, soybean (may decrease good cholesterol); butter and butter/margarine blends
Salad dressing and mayonnaise: salad dressing and mayonnaise with more than 3 grams of fat per tablespoon
Nuts: peanuts, cashews

Meats

Beef: heavily marbled or prime-grade cuts; fatty cuts like briskets, short ribs; regular ground beef
Pork: fatty cuts like spare ribs, ground pork, regular bacon*
Poultry: goose, duck, chicken, or turkey (ground with skin)

*high in sodium

Meats (*continued*)

Lamb: (all fat removed) lean cuts like leg, loin, rib
Veal: (all fat removed) all cuts except ground or cubed cutlets
Poultry: (skin removed) fresh or frozen chicken, turkey; cornish game hen; turkey ham*
Fish and Shellfish: all varieties, not breaded; canned fish packed in water
Luncheon meats and hot dogs**: Varieties with 3 grams of fat or less per ounce

Meats (*continued*)

Organ meats: liver, kidney, brain
Luncheon meats and hot dogs**: varieties with more than 3 grams of fat per ounce (includes bologna, canned luncheon meat, chopped ham, liver, sausage, regular hot dogs, and chicken or turkey hot dogs)
*Sausage**: all varieties

*high in sodium

Dear Friends,

People often ask me why I include the same general information at the beginning of all my cookbooks. If you've seen any of my other books, you'll know that my "common folk" recipes are just one part of the Healthy Exchanges picture. You know that I firmly believe—and say so whenever and wherever I can—that *Healthy Exchanges is not a diet, it's a way of life!* That's why I include the story of Healthy Exchanges in every book, because I know that the tale of my struggle to lose weight and regain my health is one that speaks to the hearts of many thousands of people. And because Healthy Exchanges is not just a collection of recipes, I always include the wisdom that I've learned from my own experiences and the knowledge of the health and cooking professionals I meet. Whether it's learning about nutrition or making shopping and cooking easier, no Healthy Exchanges book would be complete without features like "A Peek into My Pantry" or "JoAnna's Ten Commandments of Successful Cooking."

Even if you've read my other books, you might still want to skim the following chapters—you never know when I'll slip in a new bit of wisdom or suggest a new product that will make your journey to health an easier and tastier one. If you're sharing this book with a friend or family member, you'll want to make sure they read the following pages before they start stirring up the recipes.

If this is the first book of mine that you've read, I want to welcome you with all my heart to the Healthy Exchanges Family. (And, of course, I'd love to hear your comments or questions. See the back of the book for my mailing address . . . or come visit if you happen to find yourself in DeWitt, Iowa—just ask anybody for directions to Healthy Exchanges!)

JoAnna

JoAnna M. Lund and Healthy Exchanges

Food is the first invited guest to every special occasion in every family's memory scrapbook. From baptism to graduation, from weddings to wakes, food brings us together.

It wasn't always that way at our house. I used to eat alone, even when my family was there, because while they were dining on real food, I was nibbling at whatever my newest diet called for. In fact, for twenty-eight years, I called myself the diet queen of DeWitt, Iowa.

I tried every diet I ever came across, every one I could afford, and every one that found its way to my small town in eastern Iowa. I was willing to try anything that promised to "melt off the pounds," determined to deprive my body in every possible way in order to become thin at last.

I sent away for expensive "miracle" diet pills. I starved myself on the Cambridge Diet and the Bahama Diet. I gobbled diet candies, took thyroid pills, fiber pills, prescription and over-the-counter diet pills. I went to endless weight-loss support group meetings—but I somehow managed to turn healthy programs such as Overeaters Anonymous, Weight Watchers, and TOPS into unhealthy diets . . . diets I could never follow for more than a few months.

I was determined to discover something that worked long-term, but each new failure increased my desperation that I'd never find it.

I ate strange concoctions and rubbed on even stranger potions. I tried liquid diets. I agreed to be hypnotized. I tried reflexology and even had an acupressure device stuck in my ear!

Does my story sound a lot like yours? I'm not surprised. No wonder the weight-loss business is a billion-dollar industry!

Every new thing I tried seemed to work—at least at first. And losing that first five or ten pounds would get me so excited, I'd believe that this new miracle diet would, finally, get my weight off for keeps.

Inevitably, though, the initial excitement wore off. The diet's routine and boredom set in, and I quit. I shoved the pills to the back of the medicine chest, pushed the cans of powdered shake mix to the rear of the kitchen cabinets, slid all the program materials out of sight under my bed, and once more felt like a failure.

Like most dieters, I quickly gained back the weight I'd lost each time, along with a few extra "souvenir" pounds that seemed always to settle around my hips. I'd done the diet-lose-weight-gain-it-all-back "yo-yo" on the average of once a year. It's no exaggeration to say that over the years I've lost 1,000 pounds—and gained back 1,150 pounds.

Finally, at the age of forty-six, I weighed more than I'd ever imagined possible. I'd stopped believing that any diet could work for me. I drowned my sorrows in sacks of cake donuts and wondered if I'd live long enough to watch my grandchildren grow up.

Something had to change.

I had to change.

Finally, I did.

I'm over fifty now—and I'm 130 pounds less than my all-time high of close to 300 pounds. I've kept the weight off for more than seven years. I'd like to lose another 10 pounds, but I'm not obsessed about it. If it takes me two or three years to accomplish it, that's okay.

What I *do* care about is never saying hello again to any of those unwanted pounds I said good-bye to!

How did I jump off the roller coaster I was on? For one thing, I finally stopped looking to food to solve my emotional problems. But what really shook me up—and got me started on the path that changed my life—was Operation Desert Storm in early 1991. I sent three children off to the Persian Gulf war—my son-in-law, Matt, a medic in Special Forces; my daughter, Becky, a full-time college student and member of a medical unit in the Army Reserve; and my son James, a member of the Inactive Army Reserve, reactivated as a chemicals expert.

Somehow, knowing that my children were putting their lives on the line got me thinking about my own mortality—and I knew in my heart the last thing they needed while they were overseas was to get a letter from home saying that their mother was ill because of a food-related problem.

The day I drove the third child to the airport to leave for Saudi Arabia, something happened to me that would change my life for the better—and forever. I stopped praying my constant prayer as a professional dieter, which was simply "Please, God, let me lose ten pounds by Friday." Instead, I began praying, "God, please help me not to be a burden to my kids and my family." I quit praying for what I wanted and started praying for what I needed—and in the process my prayers were answered. I couldn't keep the kids safe—that was out of my hands—but I could try to get healthier to better handle the stress of it. It was the least I could do on the homefront.

That quiet prayer was the beginning of the new JoAnna Lund. My initial goal was not to lose weight or create healthy recipes. I only wanted to become healthier for my kids, my husband, and myself.

Each of my children returned safely from the Persian Gulf war. But something didn't come back—the 130 extra pounds I'd been lugging around for far too long. I'd finally accepted the truth after all those agonizing years of suffering through on-again, off-again dieting.

There are no "magic" cures in life.

No "miracle" potion, pill, or diet will make unwanted pounds disappear.

I found something better than magic, if you can believe it. When I turned my weight and health dilemma over to God for guidance, a new JoAnna Lund and Healthy Exchanges were born.

I discovered a new way to live my life—and uncovered an unexpected talent for creating easy "common folk" healthy recipes and sharing my commonsense approach to healthy living. I learned that I could motivate others to change their lives and adopt a positive outlook. I began publishing cookbooks and a monthly food newsletter, and speaking to groups all over the country.

I like to say, *"When life handed me a lemon, not only did I make healthy, tasty lemonade, I wrote the recipe down!"*

What I finally found was not a quick fix or a short-term diet, but a great way to live well for a lifetime.

I want to share it with you.

Food Exchanges and Weight Loss Choices™

If you've ever been on one of the national weight-loss programs like Weight Watchers or Diet Center, you've already been introduced to the concept of measured portions of different food groups that make up your daily food plan. If you are not familiar with such a system of weight-loss choices or exchanges, here's a brief explanation. (If you want or need more detailed information, you can write to the American Dietetic Association or the American Diabetes Association for comprehensive explanations.)

The idea of food exchanges is to divide foods into basic food groups. The foods in each group are measured in servings that have comparable values. These groups include Proteins/Meats, Breads/Starches, Fruits, Vegetables, Skim Milk, Fats, Free Foods, and Optional Calories.

Each choice or exchange included in a particular group has about the same number of calories and a similar carbohydrate, protein, and fat content as the other foods in that group. Because any food on a particular list can be "exchanged" for any other food in that group, it makes sense to call the food groups *exchanges* or *choices*.

I like to think we are also "exchanging" bad habits and food choices for good ones!

By using Weight Loss Choices or exchanges you can choose from a variety of foods without having to calculate the nutrient value of each one. This makes it easier to include a wide variety of foods in your daily menus and gives you the opportunity to tailor your choices to your unique appetite.

If you want to lose weight, you should consult your physician or other weight-control expert regarding the number of servings that would be best for you from each food group. Since men generally require more calories than women, and since the requirements for growing children and teenagers differ from those of adults, the right number of exchanges for any one person is a personal decision.

I have included a suggested plan of weight-loss choices in the pages following the exchange lists. It's a program I used to lose 130 pounds, and it's the one I still follow today.

(If you are a diabetic or have been diagnosed with heart problems, it is best to meet with your physician before using this or any other food program or recipe collection.)

Food Group Weight Loss Choices/ Exchanges

Not all food group exchanges are alike. The ones that follow are for anyone who's interested in weight loss or maintenance. If you are a diabetic, you should check with your health-care provider or dietitian to get the information you need to help you plan your diet. Diabetic exchanges are calculated by the American Diabetic Association, and information about them is provided in *The Diabetic's Healthy Exchanges Cookbook* (Perigee Books).

Every Healthy Exchanges recipe provides calculations in three ways:

- Weight Loss Choices/Exchanges

- Calories, Fat, Protein, Carbohydrates, and Fiber in grams, and Sodium and Calcium in milligrams

- Diabetic Exchanges calculated for me by a Registered Dietitian

Healthy Exchanges recipes can help you eat well and recover your health, whatever your health concerns may be. Please take a few minutes to review the exchange lists and the suggestions that follow on how to count them. You have lots of great eating in store for you!

Proteins

Meat, poultry, seafood, eggs, cheese, and legumes. One exchange of Protein is approximately 60 calories. Examples of one Protein choice or exchange:

> 1 ounce cooked weight of lean meat, poultry, or seafood
> 2 ounces white fish
> 1½ ounces 97% fat-free ham
> 1 egg (limit to no more than 4 per week)
> ¼ cup egg substitute
> 3 egg whites
> ¾ ounce reduced-fat cheese
> ½ cup fat-free cottage cheese
> 2 ounces cooked or ¾ ounce uncooked dry beans
> 1 tablespoon peanut butter (also count 1 fat exchange)

Breads

Breads, crackers, cereals, grains, and starchy vegetables. One exchange of Bread is approximately 80 calories. Examples of one Bread choice or exchange:

> 1 slice bread or 2 slices reduced-calorie bread (40 calories or less)
> 1 roll, any type (1 ounce)
> ½ cup cooked pasta or ¾ ounce uncooked (scant ½ cup)
> ½ cup cooked rice or 1 ounce uncooked (⅓ cup)
> 3 tablespoons flour
> ¾ ounce cold cereal
> ½ cup cooked hot cereal or ¾ ounce uncooked (2 tablespoons)
> ½ cup corn (kernels or cream style) or peas
> 4 ounces white potato, cooked, or 5 ounces uncooked
> 3 ounces sweet potato, cooked, or 4 ounces uncooked
> 3 cups air-popped popcorn
> 7 fat-free crackers (¾ ounce)
> 3 (2½-inch squares) graham crackers
> 2 (¾-ounce) rice cakes or 6 mini rice cakes
> 1 tortilla, any type (6-inch diameter)

Fruits

All fruits and fruit juices. One exchange of Fruit is approximately 60 calories. Examples of one Fruit choice or exchange:

1 small apple or ½ cup slices
1 small orange
½ medium banana
¾ cup berries (except strawberries and cranberries)
1 cup strawberries or cranberries
½ cup canned fruit, packed in fruit juice or rinsed well
2 tablespoons raisins
1 tablespoon spreadable fruit spread
½ cup apple juice (4 fluid ounces)
½ cup orange juice (4 fluid ounces)
½ cup applesauce

Vegetables

All fresh, canned, or frozen vegetables other than the starchy vegetables. One exchange of Vegetable is approximately 30 calories. Examples of one Vegetable choice or exchange:

½ cup vegetable
¼ cup tomato sauce
1 medium fresh tomato
½ cup vegetable juice

Skim Milk

Milk, buttermilk, and yogurt. One exchange of Skim Milk is approximately 90 calories. Examples of one Skim Milk choice or exchange:

1 cup skim milk
½ cup evaporated skim milk
1 cup low-fat buttermilk
¾ cup plain fat-free yogurt
⅓ cup nonfat dry milk powder

Fats

Margarine, mayonnaise, vegetable oils, salad dressings, olives, and nuts. One exchange of Fat is approximately 40 calories. Examples of one Fat choice or exchange:

> 1 teaspoon margarine or 2 teaspoons reduced-calorie margarine
> 1 teaspoon butter
> 1 teaspoon vegetable oil
> 1 teaspoon mayonnaise or 2 teaspoons reduced-calorie mayonnaise
> 1 teaspoon peanut butter
> 1 ounce olives
> ¼ ounce pecans or walnuts

Free Foods

Foods that do not provide nutritional value but are used to enhance the taste of foods are included in the Free Foods group. Examples of these are spices, herbs, extracts, vinegar, lemon juice, mustard, Worcestershire sauce, and soy sauce. Cooking sprays and artificial sweeteners used in moderation are also included in this group. However, you'll see that I include the caloric value of artificial sweeteners in the Optional Calories of the recipes.

You may occasionally see a recipe that lists "free food" as part of the portion. According to the published exchange lists, a free food contains fewer than 20 calories per serving. Two or three servings per day of free foods/drinks are usually allowed in a meal plan.

Optional Calories

Foods that do not fit into any other group but are used in moderation in recipes are included in Optional Calories. Foods that are counted in this way include sugar-free gelatin and puddings, fat-free mayonnaise and dressings, reduced-calorie whipped toppings, reduced-calorie syrups and jams, chocolate chips, coconut, and canned broth.

Sliders™

These are 80 Optional Calorie increments that do not fit into any particular category. You can choose which food group to *slide* these into. It is wise to limit this selection to approximately three to four per day to ensure the best possible nutrition for your body while still enjoying an occasional treat.

Sliders™ may be used in either of the following ways:

1. If you have consumed all your Protein, Bread, Fruit, or Skim Milk Weight Loss Choices for the day, and you want to eat additional foods from those food groups, you simply use a Slider. It's what I call "healthy horse trading." Remember that Sliders may not be traded for choices in the Vegetables or Fats food groups.

2. Sliders may also be deducted from your Optional Calories for the day or week. ¼ Slider equals 20 Optional Calories; ½ Slider equals 40 Optional Calories; ¾ Slider equals 60 Optional Calories; and 1 Slider equals 80 Optional Calories.

Healthy Exchanges® Weight Loss Choices™

My original Healthy Exchanges program of Weight Loss Choices™ was based on an average daily total of 1,400 to 1,600 calories per day. That was what I determined was right for my needs, and for those of most women. Because men require additional calories (about 1,600 to 1,900), here are my suggested plans for women and men. *(If you require more or fewer calories, please revise this plan to meet your individual needs.)*

Each day, women should plan to eat:

2 Skim Milk servings, 90 calories each
2 Fat servings, 40 calories each
3 Fruit servings, 60 calories each

4 Vegetable servings or more, 30 calories each
5 Protein servings, 60 calories each
5 Bread servings, 80 calories each

Each day, men should plan to eat:

2 Skim Milk servings, 90 calories each
4 Fat servings, 40 calories each
3 Fruit servings, 60 calories each
4 Vegetable servings or more, 30 calories each
6 Protein servings, 60 calories each
7 Bread servings, 80 calories each

Young people should follow the program for Men but add 1 Skim Milk serving for a total of 3 servings.

You may also choose to add up to 100 Optional Calories per day, and up to 21 to 28 Sliders per week at 80 calories each. If you choose to include more Sliders in your daily or weekly totals, deduct those 80 calories from your Optional Calorie "bank."

A word about **Sliders™**: These are to be counted toward your totals after you have used your allotment of choices of Skim Milk, Protein, Bread, and Fruit for the day. By "sliding" an additional choice into one of these groups, you can meet your individual needs for that day. Sliders are especially helpful when traveling, stressed-out, or eating out, or for special events. I often use mine so I can enjoy my favorite Healthy Exchanges desserts. Vegetables are not to be counted as Sliders. Enjoy as many Vegetable Choices as you need to feel satisfied. Because we want to limit our fat intake to moderate amounts, additional Fat Choices should not be counted as Sliders. If you choose to include more fat on an *occasional* basis, count the extra choices as Optional Calories.

Keep a daily food diary of your Weight Loss Choices, checking off what you eat as you go. If at the end of the day your required selections are not 100 percent accounted for but you have done the best you can, go to bed with a clear conscience. There will be days when you have ¼ Fruit or ½ Bread left over. What are you going to do—eat two slices of an orange or half a slice of bread and throw the rest out? I always say, "Nothing in life comes out exact." Just do the best you can . . . *the best you can.*

Try to drink at least eight 8-ounce glasses of water a day. Water truly is the "nectar" of good health.

As a little added insurance, I take a multivitamin each day. It's not essential, but if my day's worth of well-planned meals "bites the dust" when unexpected events intrude on my regular routine, my body still gets its vital nutrients.

The calories listed in each group of Choices are averages. Some choices within each group may be higher or lower, so it's important to select a variety of different foods instead of eating the same three or four all the time.

Use your Optional Calories! They are what I call "life's little extras." They make all the difference in how you enjoy your food and appreciate the variety available to you. Yes, we can get by without them, but do you really want to? Keep in mind that you should be using all your daily Weight Loss Choices first to ensure you are getting the basics of good nutrition. But I guarantee that Optional Calories will keep you from feeling deprived—and help you reach your weight-loss goals.

Sodium, Fat, Cholesterol, and Processed Foods

Are Healthy Exchanges ingredients really healthy?

When I first created Healthy Exchanges, many people asked about sodium, about whether it was necessary to calculate the percentage of fat, saturated fat, and cholesterol in a healthy diet, and about my use of processed foods in many recipes. I researched these questions as I was developing my program, so you can feel confident about using the recipes and food plan.

Sodium

Most people consume more sodium than their bodies need. The American Heart Association and the American Diabetes Association recommend limiting daily sodium intake to no more than 3,000 milligrams per day. If your doctor suggests you limit your sodium even more, then *you really must read labels.*

Sodium is an essential nutrient and should not be completely eliminated. It helps to regulate blood volume and is needed for normal daily muscle and nerve functions. Most of us, however, have no trouble getting "all we need" and then some.

As with everything else, moderation is my approach. I rarely ever have salt on my list as an added ingredient. But if you're especially sodium-sensitive, make the right choices for you—and save high-sodium foods such as sauerkraut for an occasional treat.

I use lots of spices to enhance flavors, so you won't notice the absence of salt. In the few cases where it is used, salt is vital for the success of the recipe, so please don't omit it.

When I do use an ingredient high in sodium, I try to compensate by using low-sodium products in the remainder of the recipe. Many fat-free products are a little higher in sodium to make up for any loss of flavor that disappeared along with the fat. But when I take advantage of these fat-free, higher-sodium products, I stretch that ingredient within the recipe, lowering the amount of sodium per serving. A good example is my use of fat-free and reduced-sodium canned soups. While the suggested number of servings per can is two, I make sure my final creation serves at least four and sometimes six. So the soup's sodium has been "watered down" from one-third to one-half of the original amount.

Even if you don't have to watch your sodium intake for medical reasons, using moderation is another "healthy exchange" to make on your own journey to good health.

Fat Percentages

We've been told that 30 percent is the magic number—that we should limit fat intake to 30 percent or less of our total calories. It's good advice, and I try to have a weekly average of 15 percent to 25 percent myself. I believe any less than 15 percent is really just another restrictive diet that won't last. And more than 25 percent on a regular basis is too much of a good thing.

When I started listing fat grams along with calories in my recipes, I was tempted to include the percentage of calories from fat. After all, in the vast majority of my recipes, that percentage is well below 30 percent This even includes my pie recipes that allow you a realistic serving instead of many "diet" recipes that tell you a serving is 1/12 of a pie.

Figuring fat grams is easy enough. Each gram of fat equals 9 calories. Multiply fat grams by 9, then divide that number by the total calories to get the percentage of calories from fat.

So why don't I do it? After consulting four registered dietitians for advice, I decided to omit this information. They felt that it's too easy for people to become obsessed by that 30 percent figure, which is after all supposed to be a percentage of total calories over the course of a day or a week. We mustn't feel we can't include a healthy ingredient such as pecans or olives in one recipe just because, on its own, it has more than 30 percent of its calories from fat.

An example of this would be a casserole made with 90 percent lean red meat. Most of us benefit from eating red meat in moderation, as it provides iron and niacin in our diets, and also makes life more enjoyable for us and those who eat with us. If we *only* look at the percentage of calories from fat in a serving of this one dish, which might be as high as 40 to 45 percent, we might choose not to include this recipe in our weekly food plan.

The dietitians suggested that it's important to consider the total picture when making such decisions. As long as your overall food plan keeps fat calories to 30 percent, it's all right to enjoy an occasional dish that is somewhat higher in fat content. Healthy foods I include in **MODERATION** include 90 percent lean red meat, olives, and nuts. I don't eat these foods every day, and you may not either. But occasionally, in a good recipe, they make all the difference in the world between just getting by (deprivation) and truly enjoying your food.

Remember, the goal is eating in a healthy way so you can enjoy and live well the rest of your life.

Saturated Fats and Cholesterol

You'll see that I don't provide calculations for saturated fats or cholesterol amounts in my recipes. It's for the simple and yet not so simple reason that accurate, up-to-date, brand-specific information can be difficult to obtain from food manufacturers, especially since the way in which they produce food is rapidly changing. But once more I've consulted with registered dietitians and other professionals and found that because I use only a few products that are high in saturated fat, and use them in such limited quantities, my recipes are suitable for patients concerned about controlling or lowering cholesterol. You'll also find that whenever I do use one of these ingredients *in moderation*, everything else in the recipe, and in the meals my family and I enjoy, is low in fat.

Processed Foods

Just what is processed food, anyway? What do I mean by the term "processed foods," and why do I use them, when the "purest" recipe developers in Recipe Land consider them "pedestrian" and won't ever use something from a box, container, or can? A letter I received and a passing statement from a stranger made me reflect on what I mean when I refer to processed foods, and helped me reaffirm why I use them in my "common folk" healthy recipes.

If you are like the vast millions who agree with me, then I'm not sharing anything new with you. And if you happen to disagree, that's okay, too.

A few months go, a woman sent me several articles from various "whole food" publications and wrote that she was wary of processed foods, and wondered why I used them in my recipes. She then scribbled on the bottom of her note, "Just how healthy is Healthy Exchanges?" Then, a few weeks later, during a chance visit at a public food event with a very pleasant woman, I was struck by how we all have our own definitions of what processed foods are. She shared with me, in a somewhat self-righteous manner, that she *never* uses processed foods. She only cooked with fresh fruits and vegetables, she told me. Then later she said that she used canned reduced-fat soups all the time! Was her definition different than mine, I wondered? Soup in a can, whether it's reduced in fat or not, still meets my definition of a processed food.

So I got out a copy of my book *HELP: Healthy Exchanges Lifetime Plan* and reread what I had written back then about processed foods. Nothing in my definition had changed since I wrote that section. I still believe that healthy processed foods, such as canned soups, prepared piecrusts, sugar-free instant puddings, fat-free sour cream, and frozen whipped topping, when used properly, all have a place as ingredients in healthy recipes.

I never use an ingredient that hasn't been approved by either the American Diabetic Association, the American Dietetic Association, or the American Heart Association. Whenever I'm in doubt, I send for their position papers, then ask knowledgeable registered dietitians to explain those papers to me in layman's language. I've been assured by all of them that the sugar- and fat-free products I use in my recipes are indeed safe.

If you don't agree, nothing I can say or write will convince you otherwise. But, if you've been using the healthy processed foods and have been concerned about the almost daily hoopla you hear about yet another product that's going to be the doom of all of us, then just stick with reason. For every product on the grocery shelves, there are those who want you to buy it and there are those who don't, *because they want you to buy their products instead.* So we have to learn to sift the fact from the fiction. Let's take sugar substitutes, for example. In making your own evaluations, you should be skeptical about any information provided by the sugar substitute manufacturers, because they have a vested interest in our buying their products. Likewise, ignore any information provided by the sugar industry, because they have a vested interest in our *not* buying sugar substitutes. Then, if you aren't sure if you can really trust the government or any of its agencies, toss out their data, too. That leaves the three associations I mentioned above. Do you think any of them would say a product is safe if it isn't? Or say a product isn't safe when it is? They have nothing to gain or lose, *other than their integrity,* if they intentionally try to mislead us. That's why I only go to these associations for information concerning healthy processed foods.

I certainly don't recommend that everything we eat should come from a can, box, or jar. I think the best of all possible worlds is to start with the basics: grains such as rice, pasta, or corn. Then, for example, add some raw vegetables and extra-lean meat such as poultry, fish, beef, or pork. Stir in some healthy canned soup or tomato sauce, and you'll end up with something that is not only healthy but tastes so good, everyone from toddlers to great-grandparents will want to eat it!

I've never been in favor of spraying everything we eat with chemicals, and I don't believe that all our foods should come out of packages. But I do think we should use the best available healthy processed foods to make cooking easier and food taste better. I take advantage of the good-tasting low-fat and low-sugar products found in any grocery store. My recipes are created for busy people like me, people who want to eat healthily and economically but who still want the food to satisfy their taste buds. I don't expect anyone to visit out-of-the-way health food stores or find the time to cook beans from scratch—*because I don't!* Most of you can't grow fresh food in the backyard and many of you may not have access to farmers' markets or large supermarkets. I want to help you figure out realistic ways to make healthy eating a reality *wherever you live*, or you will not stick to a healthy lifestyle for long.

So if you've been swayed (by individuals or companies with vested interests or hidden agendas) into thinking that all processed foods are bad for you, you may want to reconsider your position. Or if you've been fooling yourself into believing that you *never* use processed foods but regularly reach for that healthy canned soup, stop playing games with yourself—you are using processed foods in a healthy way. And, if you're like me and use healthy processed foods in *moderation*, don't let anyone make you feel ashamed about including these products in your healthy lifestyle. Only *you* can decide what's best for *you* and your family's needs.

Part of living a healthy lifestyle is making those decisions and then getting on with life. Congratulations on choosing to live a healthy lifestyle, and let's celebrate together by sharing a piece of Healthy Exchanges pie that I've garnished with Cool Whip Lite!

JoAnna's Ten Commandments of Successful Cooking

A very important part of any journey is knowing where you are going and the best way to get there. If you plan and prepare before you start to cook, you should reach mealtime with foods to write home about!

1. **Read the entire recipe from start to finish** and be sure you understand the process involved. Check that you have all the equipment you will need *before* you begin.

2. **Check the ingredient list** and be sure you have *everything* and in the amounts required. Keep cooking sprays handy—though they're not listed as ingredients, I use them all the time (just a quick squirt!).

3. **Set out *all* the ingredients and equipment needed** to prepare the recipe on the counter near you *before* you start. Remember that old saying *A stitch in time saves nine?* It applies in the kitchen, too.

4. **Do as much advance preparation as possible** before actually cooking. Chop, cut, grate, or do whatever is needed to prepare the ingredients and have them ready before you start to mix. Turn the oven on at least ten minutes before putting food in to bake, to allow the oven to preheat to the proper temperature.

5. **Use a kitchen timer** to tell you when the cooking or bak-

ing time is up. Because stove temperatures vary slightly by manufacturer, you may want to set your timer for five minutes less than the suggested time just to prevent overcooking. Check the progress of your dish at that time, then decide if you need the additional minutes or not.

6. **Measure carefully.** Use glass measures for liquids and metal or plastic cups for dry ingredients. My recipes are based on standard measurements. Unless I tell you it's a scant or full cup, measure the cup level.

7. **For best results, follow the recipe instructions exactly.** Feel free to substitute ingredients that *don't tamper* with the basic chemistry of the recipe, but be sure to leave key ingredients alone. For example, you could substitute sugar-free instant chocolate pudding for sugar-free instant butterscotch pudding, but if you use a six-serving package when a four-serving package is listed in the ingredients, or you use instant when cook-and-serve is required, you won't get the right result.

8. **Clean up as you go.** It is much easier to wash a few items at a time than to face a whole counter of dirty dishes later. The same is true for spills on the counter or floor.

9. **Be careful about doubling or halving a recipe**. Though many recipes can be altered successfully to serve more or fewer people, *many cannot.* This is especially true when it comes to spices and liquids. If you try to double a recipe that calls for 1 teaspoon pumpkin pie spice, for example, and you double the spice, you may end up with a too-spicy taste. I usually suggest increasing spices or liquid by 1½ times when doubling a recipe. If it tastes a little bland to you, you can increase the spice to 1¾ times the original amount the next time you prepare the dish. Remember: You can always add more, but you can't take it out after it's stirred in.

The same is true with liquid ingredients. If you wanted to **triple** a recipe like my **Italian Macaroni and Beans** because you were planning to serve a crowd, you might think you should use three times as much of every ingredient. Don't, or you could end up with Italian Macaroni and Beans Soup! The original recipe calls for 1¾ cups of chunky tomato sauce, so I'd suggest using 3½ cups when you **triple** the recipe (or 2¾ cups if you **double** it). You'll still have a good-tasting dish that won't run all over the plate.

10. **Write your reactions next to each recipe once you've served it.**

Yes, that's right, I'm giving you permission to write in this book. It's yours, after all. Ask yourself: Did everyone like it? Did you have to add another half teaspoon of chili seasoning to please your family, who like to live on the spicier side of the street? You may even want to rate the recipe on a scale of 1★ to 4★, depending on what you thought of it. (Four stars would be the top rating—and I hope you'll feel that way about many of my recipes.) Jotting down your comments while they are fresh in your mind will help you personalize the recipe to your own taste the next time you prepare it.

My Best Healthy Exchanges Tips and Tidbits

Measurements, General Cooking Tips, and Basic Ingredients

Sugar Substitutes

The word **moderation** best describes **my use of fats, sugar substitutes,** and **sodium** in these recipes. Wherever possible, I've used cooking spray for sautéing and for browning meats and vegetables. I also use reduced-calorie margarine and no-fat mayonnaise and salad dressings. Lean ground turkey *or* ground beef can be used in the recipes. Just be sure whatever you choose is at least *90 percent lean.*

I've also included **small amounts of sugar and brown sugar substitutes as the sweetening agent** in many of the recipes. I don't drink a hundred cans of soda a day or eat enough artificially sweetened foods in a 24-hour time period to be troubled by sugar substitutes. But if this is a concern of yours and you *do not* need to watch your sugar intake, you can always replace the sugar substitutes with processed sugar and the sugar-free products with regular ones.

I created my recipes knowing they would also be used by hypoglycemics, diabetics, and those concerned about triglycerides. If you choose to use sugar instead, be sure to count the additional calories.

A word of caution when cooking with **sugar substitutes**: Use **saccharin**-based sweeteners when **heating or baking**. In recipes that **don't require heat, Aspartame** (known as Nutrasweet) works well in uncooked dishes but leaves an aftertaste in baked products.

Pan Sizes

I'm often asked why I use an **8-by-8-inch baking dish** in my recipes. It's for portion control. If the recipe says it serves 4, just cut down the center, turn the dish, and cut again. Like magic, there's your serving. Also, if this is the only recipe you are preparing requiring an oven, the square dish fits into a tabletop toaster oven easily and energy can be conserved.

To make life even easier, **whenever a recipe calls for ounce measurements** (other than raw meats), I've included the closest cup equivalent. I need to use my scale daily when creating recipes, so I've measured for you at the same time.

Freezing Leftovers

Most of the recipes are for **4 to 6 servings**. If you don't have that many to feed, do what I do: freeze individual portions. Then all you have to do is choose something from the freezer and take it to work for lunch or have your evening meals prepared in advance for the week. In this way, I always have something on hand that is both good to eat and good for me.

Unless a recipe includes hard-boiled eggs, cream cheese, mayonnaise, or a raw vegetable or fruit, **the leftovers should freeze well**. (I've marked recipes that freeze well with the symbol of a **snowflake ❄.**) This includes most of the cream pies. Divide any recipe up into individual servings and freeze for your own "TV" dinners.

Another good idea is **cutting leftover pie into individual pieces and freezing each one separately** in a small Ziploc freezer bag. Then the next time you want to thaw a piece of pie for yourself, you don't have to thaw the whole pie. This is great for brown-bag lunches, too. Just pull a piece out of the freezer on your way to work and by lunchtime you will have a wonderful dessert waiting for you.

Unless I specify **"covered" for simmering or baking,** prepare my recipes **uncovered**. Occasionally you will read a recipe that asks you to cover a dish for a time, then to uncover, so read the directions carefully to avoid confusion—and to get the best results.

Cooking Spray

Low-fat cooking spray is another blessing in a Healthy Exchanges kitchen. It's currently available in three flavors:

- **OLIVE-OIL FLAVORED** when cooking Mexican, Italian, or Greek dishes
- **BUTTER FLAVORED** when the hint of butter is desired
- **REGULAR** for everything else.

A quick spray of butter flavored makes air-popped popcorn a low-fat taste treat, or try it as a butter substitute on steaming-hot corn on the cob. One light spray of the skillet when browning meat will convince you that you're using "old-fashioned fat," and a quick coating of the casserole dish before you add the ingredients will make serving easier and cleanup quicker.

Miscellaneous Ingredients/Tips

I use reduced-sodium **canned chicken broth** in place of dry bouillon to lower the sodium content. The intended flavor is still present in the prepared dish. As a reduced-sodium beef broth is not currently available (at least not in DeWitt, Iowa), I use the canned regular beef broth. The sodium content is still lower than regular dry bouillon.

Whenever **cooked rice or pasta** is an ingredient, follow the package directions, but eliminate the salt and/or margarine called for. This helps lower the sodium and fat content. It tastes just fine; trust me on this.

Here's another tip: When **cooking rice or noodles**, why not cook extra "for the pot"? After you use what you need, store leftover rice in a covered container (where it will keep for a couple of days). With noodles like spaghetti or macaroni, first rinse and drain as usual, then measure out what you need. Put the leftovers in a bowl, cover with water, then store in the refrigerator, covered, until they're needed. Then, measure out what you need, rinse and drain them, and they're ready to go.

Does your **pita bread** often tear before you can make a sandwich? Here's my tip to make them open easily: cut the bread in half, put the halves in the microwave for about 15 seconds, and they will open up by themselves. *Voilà!*

When **chunky salsa** is listed as an ingredient, I leave the degree of "heat" up to your personal taste. In our house, I'm considered a wimp. I go for the "mild" while Cliff prefers "extra-hot." How do we compromise? I prepare the recipe with mild salsa because he can always add a spoonful or two of the hotter version to his serving, but I can't enjoy the dish if it's too spicy for me.

Milk and Yogurt

Take it from me—nonfat dry milk powder is great! I *do not* use it for drinking, but I *do* use it for cooking. Three good reasons why:

(1) It is very **inexpensive**.

(2) It does not **sour** because you use it only as needed. Store the box in your refrigerator or freezer and it will keep almost forever.

(3) You can easily **add extra calcium** to just about any recipe without added liquid. I consider nonfat dry milk powder one of Mother Nature's modern-day miracles of convenience. But do purchase a good national name brand (I like Carnation), and keep it fresh by proper storage.

In many of my pies and puddings, I use nonfat dry milk powder and water instead of skim milk. Usually I call for ⅔ cup nonfat dry milk powder and 1¼ to 1½ cups water or liquid. This way I can get the nutrients of two cups of milk, but much less liquid, and the end result is much creamier. Also, the recipe sets up quicker, usually in 5 minutes or less. So if someone knocks at your door unexpectedly at mealtime, you can quickly throw a pie together and enjoy it minutes later.

You can make your own "**sour cream**" by combining ¾ cup plain fat-free yogurt with ⅓ cup nonfat dry milk powder. What you did by doing this is fourfold: 1) The dry milk stabilizes the yogurt and keeps the whey from separating. 2) The dry milk slightly helps to cut the tartness of the yogurt. 3) It's still virtually fat-free. 4) The calcium has been increased by 100 percent. Isn't it great how we can make that distant relative of sour cream a first kissin' cousin by adding the nonfat dry milk powder? Or, if you place 1 cup of plain fat-free yogurt in a sieve lined with a coffee filter, and place the sieve over a small bowl and refrigerate for about 6 hours, you will end up with a very good alternative to sour cream. To **stabilize yogurt** when cooking or baking with it, just add 1 teaspoon cornstarch to every ¾ cup yogurt.

If a recipe calls for **evaporated skim milk** and you don't have any in the cupboard, make your own. For every ½ cup evaporated skim milk needed, combine ⅓ cup nonfat dry milk powder and ½ cup water. Use as you would evaporated skim milk.

You can also make your own **sugar-free and fat-free sweetened condensed milk** at home. Combine 1⅓ cups nonfat dry milk powder and ½ cup cold water in a 2-cup glass measure. Cover and microwave on HIGH until mixture is hot but *not* boiling. Stir in ½ cup Sprinkle Sweet or Sugar Twin. Cover and refrigerate at least 4 hours. This mixture will keep for up to two weeks in the refrigerator. Use in just about any recipe that calls for sweetened condensed milk.

For any recipe that calls for **buttermilk**, you might want to try JO's Buttermilk: Blend one cup of water and ⅔ cup dry milk powder (the nutrients of two cups of skim milk). It'll be thicker than this mixed-up milk usually is because it's doubled. Add 1 teaspoon white vinegar and stir, then let it sit for at least 10 minutes.

Soup Substitutes

One of my subscribers was looking for a way to further restrict salt intake and needed a substitute for **cream of mushroom soup**. For many of my recipes, I use Healthy Request Cream of Mushroom Soup, as it is a reduced-sodium product. The label suggests two servings per can, but I usually incorporate the soup into a recipe serving at least four. By doing this, I've reduced the sodium in the soup by half again.

But if you must restrict your sodium even more, try making my Healthy Exchanges **Creamy Mushroom Sauce**. Place 1½ cups evaporated skim milk and 3 tablespoons flour in a covered jar. Shake well and pour mixture into a medium saucepan sprayed with butter-flavored cooking spray. Add ½ cup canned sliced mushrooms, rinsed and drained. Cook over medium heat, stirring often, until mixture thickens. Add any seasonings of your choice. You can use this sauce in any recipe that calls for one 10 ¾-ounce can of cream of mushroom soup.

Why did I choose these proportions and ingredients?

- 1½ cups evaporated skim milk is the amount in one can.

- It's equal to three Skim Milk choices or exchanges.

- It's the perfect amount of liquid and flour for a medium cream sauce.

- 3 tablespoons flour is equal to one Bread/Starch choice or exchange.

- Any leftovers will reheat beautifully with a flour-based sauce but not with a cornstarch-based sauce.

- The mushrooms are one Vegetable choice or exchange.

- This sauce is virtually fat-free, sugar-free, and sodium-free.

Proteins

Eggs

I use eggs in moderation. I enjoy the real thing on an average of three to four times a week. So, my recipes are calculated on using whole eggs. However, if you choose to use egg substitute in place of the egg, the finished product will turn out just fine and the fat grams per serving will be even lower than those listed.

If you like the look, taste, and feel of **hard-boiled eggs** in salads but haven't been using them because of the cholesterol in the yolk, I have a couple of alternatives for you: 1) Pour an 8-ounce carton of egg substitute into a medium skillet sprayed with cooking spray. Cover skillet tightly and cook over low heat until substitute is just set, about 10 minutes. Remove from heat and let set, still covered, for 10 minutes more. Uncover and cool completely. Chop set mixture. This will make about 1 cup of chopped egg. 2) Even easier is to hard-boil "real eggs," toss the yolk away, and chop the white. Either way, you don't deprive yourself of the pleasure of egg in your salad.

In most recipes calling for **egg substitutes**, you can use 2 egg whites in place of the equivalent of 1 egg substitute. Just break the eggs open and toss the yolks away. I can hear some of you already saying, "But that's wasteful!" Well, take a look at the price on the egg substitute package (which usually has the equivalent of 4 eggs in it), then look at the price of a dozen eggs, from which you'd get the equivalent of 6 egg substitutes. Now, what's wasteful about that?

Meat

Whenever I include **cooked chicken** in a recipe, I use roasted white meat without skin. Whenever I include **roast beef or pork** in a recipe, I use the loin cuts because they are much leaner. However, most of the time, I do my "roasting" of all these meats at the local deli. I just ask for a chunk of their lean roasted meat, 6 or 8 ounces, and ask them not to slice it. When I get home, I cube or dice the meat and am ready to use it in my recipe. The reason I do this is threefold: 1) I'm getting just the amount I need without leftovers; 2) I don't have the expense of heating the oven; and 3) I'm not throwing away the bone, gristle, and fat I'd be cutting off the meat. Overall, it is probably cheaper to "roast" it the way I do.

Did you know that you can make an acceptable meatloaf without using egg for the binding? Just replace every egg with ¼ cup of liquid. You could use beef broth, tomato sauce, even applesauce, to name just a few. For a meatloaf to serve 6, I always use 1 pound of extra-lean ground beef or turkey, 6 tablespoons of dried fine bread crumbs, and ¼ cup of the liquid, plus anything else healthy that strikes my fancy at the time. I mix well and place the mixture in an 8-by-8-inch baking dish or 9-by-5-inch loaf pan sprayed with cooking spray. Bake uncovered at 350 degrees for 35 to 50 minutes (depending on the added ingredients). You will never miss the egg.

Any time you are **browning ground meat** for a casserole and want to get rid of almost all the excess fat, just place the uncooked meat loosely in a plastic colander. Set the colander in a glass pie plate. Place in microwave and cook on HIGH for 3 to 6 minutes (depending on the amount being browned), stirring often. Use as you would for any casserole. You can also chop up onions and brown them with the meat if you want.

Gravy

For **gravy** with all the "old time" flavor but without the extra fat, try this almost effortless way to prepare it (it's almost as easy as opening up a store-bought jar): Pour the juice off your roasted meat, then set the roast aside to "rest" for about 20 minutes. Place the juice in an uncovered cake pan or other large flat pan (we want the large air surface to speed up the cooling process), and put in the freezer until the fat congeals on top and you can skim it off. Or, if you prefer, use a skimming pitcher purchased at your kitchen gadget store. Either way, measure about 1½ cups skimmed broth and pour into a medium saucepan. Cook over medium heat until heated through, about 5 minutes. In a covered jar, combine ½ cup water or cooled potato broth with 3 tablespoons flour. Shake well. Pour flour mixture into warmed juice. Combine well using a wire whisk. Continue cooking until gravy thickens, about 5 minutes. Season with salt and pepper to taste.

Why did I use flour instead of cornstarch? Because any leftovers will reheat nicely with the flour base and would not with a cornstarch base. Also, 3 tablespoons of flour works out to 1 Bread/Starch exchange. This virtually fat-free gravy makes about 2 cups, so you could spoon about ½ cup gravy on your low-fat mashed potatoes and only have to count your gravy as ¼ Bread/Starch exchange.

Fruits and Vegetables

If you want to enjoy a **"fruit shake"** with some pizazz, just combine soda water and unsweetened fruit juice in a blender. Add crushed ice. Blend on HIGH until thick. Refreshment without guilt.

You'll see that many recipes use ordinary **canned vegetables**. They're much cheaper than reduced-sodium versions, and once you rinse and drain them, the sodium is reduced anyway. I believe in saving money wherever possible so we can afford the best fat-free and sugar-free products as they come onto the market.

All three kinds of **vegetables—fresh, frozen, and canned—** have their place in a healthy diet. My husband, Cliff, hates the taste of frozen or fresh green beans, thinks the texture is all wrong, so I use canned green beans instead. In this case, canned vegetables have their proper place when I'm feeding my husband. If someone in your family has a similar concern, it's important to respond to it so everyone can be happy and enjoy the meal.

When I use **fruits or vegetables** like apples, cucumbers, and zucchini, I wash them really well and **leave the skin on**. It provides added color, fiber, and attractiveness to any dish. And, because I use processed flour in my cooking, I like to increase the fiber in my diet by eating my fruits and vegetables in their closest-to-natural state.

To keep help **fresh fruits and veggies fresh**, just give them a quick "shower" with lemon juice. The easiest way to do this is to pour purchased lemon juice into a kitchen spray bottle and store in the refrigerator. Then, every time you use fresh fruits or vegetables in a salad or dessert, simply give them a quick spray with your "lemon spritzer." You might just be amazed by how this little trick keeps your produce from turning brown so fast.

The next time you warm canned vegetables such as carrots or green beans, drain and heat the vegetables in ¼ cup beef or chicken broth. It gives a nice variation to an old standby. Here's a simple **white sauce** for vegetables and casseroles without using added fat that can be made by spraying a medium saucepan with butter-flavored cooking spray. Place 1½ cups evaporated skim milk and 3 tablespoons flour in a covered jar. Shake well. Pour into sprayed saucepan and cook over medium heat until thick, stirring constantly. Add salt and pepper to taste. You can also add ½ cup canned drained mushrooms and/or 3 ounces (¾ cup) shredded reduced-fat cheese. Continue cooking until cheese melts.

Zip up canned or frozen green beans with **chunky salsa:** ½ cup salsa to 2 cups beans. Heat thoroughly. Chunky salsa also makes a wonderful dressing on lettuce salads. It only counts as a vegetable, so enjoy.

Another wonderful **South of the Border** dressing can be stirred up by using ½ cup of chunky salsa and ¼ cup fat-free Ranch dressing. Cover and store in your refrigerator. Use as a dressing for salads or as a topping for baked potatoes.

Delightful Dessert Ideas

Thaw **lite whipped topping** in the refrigerator overnight. Never try to force the thawing by stirring or using a microwave to soften. Stirring the topping will remove the air that gives it the lightness and texture we want, and there's not enough fat in it to survive being heated.

How can I **frost an entire pie with just ½ cup of whipped topping?** First, don't use an inexpensive brand. I use Cool Whip Lite or La Creme Lite. Make sure the topping is fully thawed. Always spread from the center to the sides using a rubber spatula. This way, ½ cup topping will literally cover an entire pie. Remember, the operative word is *frost*, not pile the entire container on top of the pie! For a special treat that tastes anything but "diet," try placing **spreadable fruit** in a container and microwave for about 15 seconds. Then pour the melted fruit spread over a serving of nonfat ice cream or frozen yogurt. One tablespoon of spreadable fruit is equal to 1 fruit serving. Some combinations to get you started are apricot over chocolate ice cream, strawberry over strawberry ice cream, or any flavor over vanilla.

Another way I use spreadable fruit is to make a delicious **topping for a cheesecake or angel food cake**. I take ½ cup fruit and ½ cup Cool Whip Lite and blend the two together with a teaspoon of coconut extract.

Here's a really **good topping** for the fall of the year. Place 1½ cups unsweetened applesauce in a medium saucepan or 4-cup glass measure. Stir in 2 tablespoons raisins, 1 teaspoon apple pie spice, and 2 tablespoons Cary's Sugar Free Maple Syrup. Cook over medium heat on stove or process on HIGH in microwave until warm. Then spoon about ½ cup warm mixture over pancakes, French toast, or fat-free and sugar-free vanilla ice cream. It's as close as you will get to guilt-free apple pie!

A quick yet tasty way to prepare **strawberries for shortcake** is to place about ¾ cup sliced strawberries, 2 tablespoons Diet Mountain Dew, and sugar substitute to equal ¼ cup sugar in a blender container. Process on BLEND until mixture is smooth. Pour mixture into bowl. Add 1¼ cups sliced strawberries and mix well. Cover and refrigerate until ready to serve with shortcake.

The next time you are making treats for the family, try using **unsweetened applesauce** for some or all of the required oil in the recipe. For instance, if the recipe calls for ½ cup cooking oil, use up to the ½ cup in applesauce. It works and most people will not even notice the difference. It's great in purchased cake mixes, but so far I haven't been able to figure out a way to deep-fat fry with it!

Another trick I often use is to include tiny amounts of "real people" food, such as coconut, but extend the flavor by using extracts. Try it—you will be surprised by how little of the real thing you can use and still feel you are not being deprived.

If you are preparing a pie filling that has ample moisture, just line **graham crackers** in the bottom of a 9-by-9-inch cake pan. Pour the filling over the top of the crackers. Cover and refrigerate until the moisture has enough time to soften the crackers. Overnight is best. This eliminates the added **fats and sugars of a piecrust.**

When **stirring fat-free cream cheese to soften it,** use only a sturdy spoon, never an electric mixer. The speed of a mixer can cause the cream cheese to lose its texture and become watery.

Did you know you can make your own **fruit-flavored yogurt?** Mix 1 tablespoon of any flavor of spreadable fruit spread with ¾ cup plain yogurt. It's every bit as tasty and much cheaper. You can also make your own **lemon yogurt** by combining 3 cups plain fat-free yogurt with 1 tub Crystal Light lemonade powder. Mix well, cover, and store in refrigerator. I think you will be pleasantly surprised by the ease, cost, and flavor of this "made from scratch" calcium-rich treat. P.S.: You can make any flavor you like by using any of the Crystal Light mixes—Cranberry? Iced Tea? You decide.

Sugar-free puddings and gelatins are important to many of my recipes, but if you prefer to avoid sugar substitutes, you could still prepare the recipes with regular puddings or gelatins. The calories would be higher, but you would still be cooking low-fat.

When a recipe calls for **chopped nuts** (and you only have whole ones), who wants to dirty the food processor just for a couple of tablespoonsful? You could try to chop them using your cutting board, but be prepared for bits and pieces to fly all over the kitchen. I use "Grandma's food processor." I take the biggest nuts I can find, put them in a small glass bowl, and chop them into chunks just the right size using a metal biscuit cutter.

If you have a **leftover muffin** and are looking for something a little different for breakfast, you can make a **"breakfast sundae."** Crumble the muffin into a cereal bowl. Sprinkle a serving of fresh fruit over it and top with a couple of tablespoons of nonfat plain yogurt sweetened with sugar substitute and your choice of extract. The thought of it just might make you jump out of bed with a smile on your face. (Speaking of muffins, did you know that if you fill the unused muffin wells with water when baking muffins, you help ensure more even baking and protect the muffin pan at the same time?) Another muffin hint: Lightly spray the inside of paper baking cups with butter-flavored cooking spray before spooning the muffin batter into them. Then you won't end up with paper clinging to your fresh-baked muffins.

The secret of making **good meringues** without sugar is to use 1 tablespoon of Sprinkle Sweet or Sugar Twin for every egg white, and a small amount of extract. Use ½ to 1 teaspoon for the batch. Almond, vanilla, and coconut are all good choices. Use the same amount of cream of tartar you usually do. Bake the meringue in the same old way. Don't think you can't have meringue pies because you can't eat sugar. You can, if you do it my way. (Remember that egg whites whip up best at room temperature.)

Homemade or Store-Bought?

I've been asked which is better for you: homemade from scratch, or purchased foods. My answer is *both!* Each has a place in a healthy lifestyle, and what that place is has everything to do with you.

Take **piecrusts**, for instance. If you love spending your spare time in the kitchen preparing foods, and you're using low-fat, low-sugar, and reasonably low-sodium ingredients, go for it! But if, like so many people, your time is limited and you've learned to read labels, you could be better off using purchased crust.

I know that when I prepare a pie (and I experiment with a couple of pies each week, because this is Cliff's favorite dessert), I use a purchased crust. Why? Mainly because I can't make a good-tasting piecrust that is lower in fat than the brands I use. Also, purchased piecrusts fit my rule of "If it takes longer to fix than to eat, forget it!"

I've checked the nutrient information for the purchased piecrusts against recipes for traditional and "diet" piecrusts, using my computer software program. The purchased crust calculated lower in both fat and calories! I have tried some low-fat and low-sugar recipes, but they just didn't spark my taste buds, or were so complicated you needed an engineering degree just to get the crust in the pie plate.

I'm very happy with the purchased piecrusts in my recipes because the finished product rarely, if ever, has more than 30 percent of total calories coming from fats. I also believe that we have to prepare foods our families and friends will eat with us on a regular basis and not feel deprived, or we've wasted time, energy, and money.

I could use a purchased "lite" **pie filling**, but instead I make my own. Here I can save both fat and sugar, and still make the filling almost as fast as opening a can. The bottom line: Know what you have to spend when it comes to both time and fat/sugar calories, then make the best decision you can for you and your family. And don't go without an occasional piece of pie because you think it isn't *necessary*. A delicious pie prepared in a healthy way is one of the simple pleasures of life. It's a little thing, but it can make all the difference between just getting by with the bare minimum and living a full and healthy lifestyle.

Many people have experimented with my tip about **substituting applesauce and artificial sweetener for butter and sugar**, but what if you aren't satisfied with the result? One woman wrote to me about a recipe for her grandmother's cookies that called for 1 cup of butter and 1½ cups of sugar. Well, any recipe that depends on as much butter and sugar as this one does is generally not a good candidate for "healthy exchanges." The original recipe needed a large quantity of fat to produce a crisp cookie just like Grandma made.

Unsweetened applesauce can be used to substitute for vegetable oil with various degrees of success, but not to replace butter, lard, or margarine. If your recipe calls for ½ cup oil or less, and it's a quick bread, muffin, or bar cookie, it should work to replace the oil with applesauce. If the recipe calls for more than ½ cup oil, then experiment with half oil, half applesauce. You've still made the recipe healthier, even if you haven't removed all the oil from it.

Another rule for healthy substitution: Up to ½ cup sugar or less can be replaced by *an artificial sweetener that can withstand the heat of baking*, like Sugar Twin or Sprinkle Sweet. If it requires more than ½ cup sugar, cut the amount needed by 75 percent and use ½ cup sugar substitute and sugar for the rest. Other options: reduce the butter and sugar by 25 percent and see if the finished product still satisfies you in taste and appearance. Or, make the cookies just like Grandma did, realizing they are part of your family's holiday tradition. Enjoy a moderate serving of a couple of cookies once or twice during the season, and just forget about them the rest of the year.

I'm sure you'll add to this list of cooking tips as you begin preparing Healthy Exchanges recipes and discover how easy it can be to adapt your own favorite recipes using these ideas and your own common sense.

A Peek into My Pantry and My Favorite Brands

Everyone asks me what foods I keep on hand and what brands I use. There are lots of good products on the grocery shelves today—many more than we dreamed about even a year or two ago. And I can't wait to see what's out there twelve months from now. The following are my staples and, where appropriate, my favorites *at this time*. I feel these products are healthier, tastier, easy to get— and deliver the most flavor for the least amount of fat, sugar, or calories. If you find others you like as well *or better,* please use them. This is only a guide to make your grocery shopping and cooking easier.

Fat-free plain yogurt (Yoplait or Dannon)
Nonfat dry milk powder (Carnation)
Evaporated skim milk (Carnation)
Skim milk
Fat-free cottage cheese
Fat-free cream cheese (Philadelphia)
Fat-free mayonnaise (Kraft)
Fat-free salad dressings (Kraft)
Fat-free sour cream (Land O Lakes)
Reduced-calorie margarine (Weight Watchers, Promise, or
  Smart Beat)
Cooking spray
  Olive-oil flavored and regular (Pam)

Butter flavored for sautéing (Weight Watchers)
Butter flavored for spritzing after cooking (I Can't Believe It's Not Butter!)
Vegetable oil (Puritan Canola Oil)
Reduced-calorie whipped topping (Cool Whip Lite or Cool Whip Free)
Sugar substitute
  if no heating is involved (Equal)
  if heating is required
    white (Sugar Twin or Sprinkle Sweet)
    brown (Brown Sugar Twin)
Sugar-free gelatin and pudding mixes (JELL-O)
Baking mix (Bisquick Reduced Fat)
Pancake mix (Aunt Jemima Reduced-Calorie)
Reduced-calorie pancake syrup (Cary's Sugar Free)
Parmesan cheese (Kraft fat-free)
Reduced-fat cheese (Kraft ⅓ Less Fat)
Shredded frozen potatoes (Mr. Dell's)
Spreadable fruit spread (Smucker's, Welch's, or Knott's Berry Farm)
Peanut butter (Peter Pan reduced-fat, Jif reduced-fat, or Skippy reduced-fat)
Chicken broth (Healthy Request)
Beef broth (Swanson)
Tomato sauce (Hunt's—plain, Italian, or chili)
Canned soups (Healthy Request)
Tomato juice (Campbell's Reduced-Sodium)
Ketchup (Heinz Light Harvest or Healthy Choice)
Purchased piecrust
  unbaked (Pillsbury—from dairy case)
  graham cracker, butter flavored, or chocolate flavored (Keebler)
Crescent rolls (Pillsbury Reduced Fat)
Pastrami and corned beef (Carl Buddig Lean)
Luncheon meats (Healthy Choice or Oscar Mayer)
Ham (Dubuque 97% fat-free and reduced-sodium or Healthy Choice)
Frankfurters and Kielbasa sausage (Healthy Choice)
Canned white chicken, packed in water (Swanson)

Canned tuna, packed in water (Chicken of the Sea)
90–95 percent lean ground turkey and beef
Soda crackers (Nabisco Fat-Free)
Reduced-calorie bread—40 calories per slice or less
Hamburger buns—80 calories each (Less)
Rice—instant, regular, brown, and wild
Instant potato flakes (Betty Crocker Potato Buds)
Noodles, spaghetti, and macaroni
Salsa (Chi Chi's Mild Chunky)
Pickle relish—dill, sweet, and hot dog
Mustard—Dijon, prepared, and spicy
Unsweetened apple juice
Unsweetened applesauce
Fruit—fresh, frozen (no sugar added), or canned in juice
Vegetables—fresh, frozen, or canned
Spices—JO's Spices
Lemon and lime juice (in small plastic fruit-shaped bottles
    found in produce section)
Instant fruit beverage mixes (Crystal Light)
Dry dairy beverage mixes (Nestlé's Quik or Swiss Miss)
Ice Cream—Wells' Blue Bunny sugar- and fat-free

The items on my shopping list are everyday foods found in just about any grocery store in America. But all are as low in fat, sugar, calories, and sodium as I can find—and still taste good! I can make any recipe in my cookbooks and newsletters as long as I have my cupboards and refrigerator stocked with these items. Whenever I use the last of any one item, I just make sure I pick up another supply the next time I'm at the store.

If your grocer does not stock these items, why not ask if they can be ordered on a trial basis? If the store agrees to do so, be sure to tell your friends to stop by, so that sales are good enough to warrant restocking the new products. Competition for shelf space is fierce, so only products that sell well stay around.

How to Read a
Healthy
Exchanges Recipe

The Healthy Exchanges Nutritional Analysis

Before using these recipes, you may wish to consult your physician or health-care provider to be sure they are appropriate for you. The information in this book is not intended to take the place of any medical advice. It reflects my experiences, studies, research, and opinions regarding healthy eating.

Each recipe includes nutritional information calculated in three ways:

> Healthy Exchanges Weight Loss Choices™ or Exchanges
> Calories, calcium, fiber, and fat grams
> Diabetic exchanges

In every Healthy Exchanges recipe, the diabetic exchanges have been calculated by a registered dietitian. All the other calculations were done by computer, using the Food Processor II software. When the ingredient listing gives more than one choice, the first ingredient listed is the one used in the recipe analysis. Due to inevitable variations in the ingredients you choose to use, the nutritional values should be considered approximate.

The annotation "(limited)" following Protein counts in some recipes indicates that consumption of whole eggs should be limited to four per week.

Please note the following symbols:

☆ This star means read the recipe's directions carefully for special instructions about **division** of ingredients.

❋ This symbol indicates **FREEZES WELL.**

The Recipes

Soups

Summer Breeze Gazpacho

There just isn't a more delicious way to get all your veggies than combining them in this colorful and freshly made salad-in-a-cup! Imagine sitting outside in your garden as the summer sun is setting and sipping this tangy treat. . . . Doesn't that sound refreshing?

● Serves 6 (1¼ cups)

> 2 cups Healthy Request tomato juice or any reduced-sodium
>   tomato juice
> 1¾ cups (one 14½-ounce can) Swanson Beef Broth
> 1 teaspoon Sugar Twin or Sprinkle Sweet
> 1½ cups chopped fresh tomatoes
> ½ cup shredded carrots
> ¼ cup finely chopped onion
> ¾ cup chopped green bell pepper
> 1 cup chopped unpeeled cucumber
> 1 cup chopped unpeeled zucchini or any summer squash
> 1 tablespoon chopped fresh parsley or 1 teaspoon dried parsley
>   flakes

In a large bowl, combine tomato juice, beef broth, and sugar substitute. Stir in tomatoes, carrots, onion, green pepper, cucumber, zucchini, and parsley. Cover and refrigerate for at least 2 hours. Stir again just before serving.

HINT: Good served with reduced-fat crackers and cheese for a cool summer meal.

Each serving equals:

HE: 2⅓ Vegetable • 6 Optional Calories

44 Calories • 0 gm Fat • 2 gm Protein •
9 gm Carbohydrate • 258 mg Sodium •
22 mg Calcium • 2 gm Fiber

DIABETIC: 2 Vegetable

Italian Tomato Noodle Soup

Why not join me on a delightful culinary journey this evening—
and prepare this delectable soup that's *delizioso* enough to appear
on the menu of your favorite Italian restaurant? Soup that gives us
such a great aroma is sure to bring your *famiglia* together at the
table! ◐ Serves 4 (scant 1½ cups)

¼ cup finely chopped onion
1 (10¾-ounce) can Healthy Request Tomato Soup
1¾ cups (one 14½-ounce can) stewed tomatoes, undrained
1 cup water
1 cup skim milk
½ cup (one 2.5-ounce jar) sliced mushrooms, drained
1½ teaspoons Italian seasoning
1¼ cups (2¼ ounces) uncooked noodles
¼ cup (¾ ounce) grated Kraft fat-free Parmesan cheese

In a large saucepan sprayed with olive oil–flavored cooking
spray, sauté onion for about 5 minutes. Add tomato soup,
undrained stewed tomatoes, water, skim milk, mushrooms, and
Italian seasoning. Mix well to combine. Stir in uncooked noodles.
Lower heat and simmer for 10 minutes or until noodles are tender.
When serving, top each bowl with 1 tablespoon Parmesan cheese.

Each serving equals:

HE: 1¼ Vegetable • ¾ Bread • ¼ Protein •
¼ Skim Milk • ½ Slider • 5 Optional Calories

194 Calories • 2 gm Fat • 7 gm Protein •
37 gm Carbohydrate • 776 mg Sodium •
149 mg Calcium • 3 gm Fiber

DIABETIC: 2 Starch • 1 Vegetable • ½ Meat

Southwestern Chicken-Cheese Soup

Cliff and I love traveling to Arizona when we can to visit our son Tommy and his wife, Angie, but sometimes we feel close to them when we savor a recipe full of the flavors of the Southwest. Mingling chicken, cheese, and corn with some splendid spices prompted Cliff to yell "Olé!" ☻ Serves 4 (1½ cups)

> 2 cups (one 16-ounce can) Healthy Request Chicken Broth
> ½ cup chunky salsa (mild, medium, or hot)
> 1 (10¾-ounce) can Healthy Request Cream of Chicken Soup
> ½ cup (one 2.5-ounce jar) sliced mushrooms, drained
> ½ cup (3 ounces) finely diced cooked chicken breast
> 1½ cups frozen whole-kernel corn, thawed
> ⅓ cup Carnation Nonfat Dry Milk Powder
> ½ cup water
> ¼ teaspoon black pepper
> ¾ cup (3 ounces) shredded Kraft reduced-fat Cheddar cheese

In a large saucepan, combine chicken broth, salsa, chicken soup, mushrooms, chicken, and corn. Bring mixture to a boil. Lower heat and simmer. Meanwhile, in a small bowl, combine dry milk powder and water. Stir milk mixture into chicken mixture. Add black pepper and Cheddar cheese. Mix well to combine. Continue simmering for 5 minutes or until cheese melts, stirring often.

HINTS: 1. If you don't have leftovers, purchase a chunk of cooked chicken breast from your local deli.
2. Thaw corn by placing in a colander and rinsing under hot water for one minute.

Each serving equals:

HE: 1¾ Protein • ¾ Bread • ½ Vegetable •
¼ Skim Milk • ½ Slider • 13 Optional Calories

259 Calories • 7 gm Fat • 23 gm Protein •
26 gm Carbohydrate • 987 mg Sodium •
276 mg Calcium • 2 gm Fiber

DIABETIC: 1½ Meat • 1½ Starch • ½ Vegetable

Broccoli Chicken-Noodle Soup ❄

Broccoli has so many health benefits, it's a great choice for anyone interested in living a healthier lifestyle. This tasty soup was greeted warmly by just about all my recipe testers, except my husband, Cliff, of course, who still doesn't care for this particular "B" vegetable!

● Serves 6 (1¼ cups)

> 2 cups (one 16-ounce can) Healthy Request Chicken Broth
> 1 cup water
> 1¾ cups (3 ounces) uncooked noodles
> 3 cups frozen chopped broccoli
> 1 (10¾-ounce) can Healthy Request Cream of Chicken Soup
> 1½ cups (one 12-fluid-ounce can) Carnation Evaporated Skim Milk
> 1 cup (5 ounces) diced cooked chicken breast
> ¼ teaspoon lemon pepper
> ¾ cup (3 ounces) shredded Kraft reduced-fat Cheddar cheese

In a slow cooker container, combine chicken broth, water, uncooked noodles, and broccoli. Cover and cook on LOW for 3 hours. Stir in chicken soup, evaporated skim milk, chicken, and lemon pepper. Cover and continue cooking on LOW for 1 hour. Stir in Cheddar cheese. Serve at once.

HINT: If you don't have leftovers, purchase a chunk of cooked chicken breast from your local deli.

Each serving equals:

HE: 1½ Protein • 1 Vegetable • ⅔ Bread •
½ Skim Milk • ¼ Slider • 15 Optional Calories

220 Calories • 4 gm Fat • 21 gm Protein •
25 gm Carbohydrate • 806 mg Sodium •
320 mg Calcium • 2 gm Fiber

DIABETIC: 1½ Meat • 1 Vegetable • 1 Starch •
½ Skim Milk

Chicken Pot Soup

❄

Remember when a beloved United States president promised Americans "a chicken in every pot"? I bet he'd cast his vote for this truly creamy and chicken-y soup—and it'll win in a landslide at your house. (My son Tommy told me this soup was easy for a college boy to fix—and tasted like a chicken pot pie.)

○ Serves 4 (1 full cup)

> 1 (10¾-ounce) can Healthy Request Cream of Chicken Soup
> 1⅓ cups skim milk
> 1 cup (5 ounces) diced cooked chicken breast
> 1 teaspoon dried parsley flakes
> 1 cup (one 8-ounce can) peas, rinsed and drained
> 2 cups (one 16-ounce can) cut carrots, rinsed and drained

In a large saucepan, combine chicken soup, skim milk, chicken, and parsley flakes. Stir in peas and carrots. Lower heat and simmer for 10 minutes or until mixture is heated through, stirring often.

HINT: If you don't have leftovers, purchase a chunk of cooked chicken breast from your local deli.

Each serving equals:

HE: 1¼ Protein • 1 Vegetable • ½ Bread •
⅓ Skim Milk • ½ Slider • 5 Optional Calories

179 Calories • 3 gm Fat • 17 gm Protein •
21 gm Carbohydrate • 401 mg Sodium •
134 mg Calcium • 3 gm Fiber

DIABETIC: 1 Meat • 1 Vegetable • 1 Starch

Chicken Wild Rice Soup

Many people have told me they enjoy the nutty flavor of the grain called wild rice, but they're not always sure how to use it in recipes. This luscious dish features it beautifully and will make any meal feel like a special occasion!　❍　Serves 4 (1½ cups)

> 2 cups (one 16-ounce can) Healthy Request Chicken Broth
> 2 cups water
> ½ cup chopped onion
> 1 cup shredded carrots
> 1 cup sliced celery
> 1 full cup (6 ounces) diced cooked chicken breast
> 1 (10¾-ounce) can Healthy Request Cream of Mushroom Soup
> Scant 1 cup (3 ounces) uncooked instant long grain and wild rice

In a large saucepan, combine chicken broth, water, onion, carrots, and celery. Bring mixture to a boil. Stir in chicken. Lower heat, cover, and simmer for 10 minutes or until vegetables are tender. Add mushroom soup and uncooked instant wild rice. Mix well to combine. Re-cover and continue simmering for 10 minutes or until rice is tender, stirring occasionally.

HINT:　If you don't have leftovers, purchase a chunk of cooked chicken breast from your local deli.

Each serving equals:

HE: 1½ Protein • 1¼ Vegetable • ¾ Bread •
½ Slider • 9 Optional Calories

---

233 Calories • 5 gm Fat • 25 gm Protein •
22 gm Carbohydrate • 974 mg Sodium •
98 mg Calcium • 2 gm Fiber

DIABETIC: 1½ Meat • 1½ Starch • 1 Vegetable

Texas Vegetable Soup

Big on nutrition, big on flavor—in fact, just plain BIG! A healthy serving of this savory veggie soup will fill your tummy AND soothe your soul. ☻ Serves 6 (1½ cups)

16 ounces ground 90% lean
   turkey or beef
1 cup chopped onion
1 cup chopped celery
1¾ cups (one 14½-ounce can)
   Swanson Beef Broth
2 cups Healthy Request
   tomato juice or any
   reduced-sodium
   tomato juice
6 ounces (one 8-ounce can)
   red kidney beans, rinsed
   and drained

2 cups (one 16-ounce can)
   tomatoes, coarsely
   chopped and undrained
1½ cups frozen whole-kernel
   corn, thawed
1 cup frozen sliced carrots,
   thawed
1 cup frozen cut green beans,
   thawed
½ teaspoon dried minced
   garlic
1 teaspoon chili seasoning
¼ teaspoon black pepper

In a large saucepan sprayed with olive oil–flavored cooking spray, brown meat and onion. Add celery, beef broth, tomato juice, kidney beans, undrained tomatoes, corn, carrots, and green beans. Mix well to combine. Stir in garlic, chili seasoning, and black pepper. Bring mixture to a boil. Lower heat, cover, and simmer for 30 minutes, stirring occasionally.

HINT: Thaw vegetables by placing in a colander and rinsing under hot water for one minute.

Each serving equals:

HE: 2⅔ Vegetable • 2½ Protein • ½ Bread •
6 Optional Calories

239 Calories • 7 gm Fat • 19 gm Protein •
25 gm Carbohydrate • 356 mg Sodium •
45 mg Calcium • 6 gm Fiber

DIABETIC: 2 Vegetable • 2 Meat • 1 Starch

Spanish Beef and Corn Chowder ✳

On a chilly fall evening when all you really want is a bowlful of comfort, here's a soup that's amazingly easy to love. Isn't it wonderful to know that taking good care of yourself can also taste this good?   ☺   Serves 4 (1¼ cups)

> *8 ounces ground 90% lean turkey or beef*
> *½ cup finely chopped onion*
> *½ cup finely chopped green bell pepper*
> *1¾ cups (one 14½-ounce can) Swanson Beef Broth*
> *½ cup (one 2.5-ounce jar) sliced mushrooms, drained*
> *2 cups frozen whole-kernel corn, thawed*
> *1 teaspoon chili seasoning*
> *1 teaspoon dried parsley flakes*
> *1 (10¾-ounce) can Healthy Request Cream of Mushroom Soup*
> *1 cup skim milk*

In a large saucepan sprayed with butter-flavored cooking spray, brown meat, onion, and green pepper. Add beef broth, mushrooms, corn, chili seasoning, and parsley flakes. Mix well to combine. Lower heat and simmer for 10 minutes, stirring occasionally. Stir in mushroom soup and skim milk. Continue simmering about 5 minutes or until mixture is heated through, stirring often.

HINT: Thaw corn by placing in a colander and rinsing under hot water for one minute.

Each serving equals:

> HE: 1½ Protein • 1 Bread • ¾ Vegetable •
> ¼ Skim Milk • ½ Slider • 1 Optional Calorie
>
> ―――――――――――――――――――――――――――――
> 242 Calories • 6 gm Fat • 17 gm Protein •
> 30 gm Carbohydrate • 832 mg Sodium •
> 136 mg Calcium • 3 gm Fiber
> ―――――――――――――――――――――――――――――
> DIABETIC: 2 Starch • 1½ Meat

Kansas City "Beefy" Tomato Soup ❄

What could be simpler than this "super" soup, inspired by a meal we shared in Kansas City with our nephew John Benischek? If you don't have leftovers, do what I often do: stir in diced-up roasted deli meat, or even try using eight ounces of browned ground 90 percent lean turkey or beef. ☻ Serves 4 (1 full cup)

1 full cup (6 ounces) diced cooked lean roast beef
1 (10¾-ounce) can Healthy Request Tomato Soup
1¾ cups (one 15-ounce can) Hunt's Tomato Sauce
1 cup water
1 teaspoon Italian seasoning

In a medium saucepan, combine roast beef, tomato soup, tomato sauce, water, and Italian seasoning. Bring mixture to a boil. Lower heat and simmer for 10 minutes, stirring occasionally.

Hints: 1. If you don't have leftovers, purchase a chunk of cooked lean roast beef from your local deli, or use packaged 97% fat-free roast beef deli slices.
2. 8 ounces browned ground 90% lean turkey or beef may be used in place of cooked roast beef.

Each serving equals:

HE: 1¾ Vegetable • 1½ Protein • ½ Slider •
5 Optional Calories

127 Calories • 3 gm Fat • 14 gm Protein •
11 gm Carbohydrate • 1,168 mg Sodium •
17 mg Calcium • 3 gm Fiber

DIABETIC: 2 Vegetable • 1½ Meat

Beef and Noodle Soup

What could be cozier than this rich and fragrant soup just brimming with noodles and beef? It's as filling as a buffet in a bowl!

☻   Serves 4 (1½ cups)

> 1 full cup (6 ounces) diced cooked lean roast beef
> ½ cup chopped onion
> 1¾ cups (one 14½-ounce can) Swanson Beef Broth
> 2¼ cups water
> ⅛ teaspoon black pepper
> ¼ teaspoon dried minced garlic
> 1¾ cups (3 ounces) uncooked noodles
> ½ cup (one 2.5-ounce jar) sliced mushrooms, drained
> 1 teaspoon dried parsley flakes

In a large saucepan sprayed with butter-flavored cooking spray, sauté roast beef and onion for 5 minutes. Add beef broth, water, black pepper, and garlic. Mix well to combine. Bring mixture to a boil. Lower heat and simmer for 10 minutes. Add uncooked noodles, mushrooms, and parsley flakes. Mix well to combine. Cover and simmer for 10 minutes or until noodles are tender.

HINT: If you don't have leftovers, purchase a chunk of cooked lean roast beef from your local deli, or use a package of Healthy Choice 97% fat-free deli slices.

Each serving equals:

> HE: 1½ Protein • 1 Bread • ½ Vegetable •
> 9 Optional Calories
>
> ---
>
> 188 Calories • 4 gm Fat • 17 gm Protein •
> 21 gm Carbohydrate • 475 mg Sodium •
> 19 mg Calcium • 2 gm Fiber
>
> ---
>
> DIABETIC: 1½ Meat • 1½ Starch

James's Quick and Thick Chili ❄

No time to cook? Lots of hungry baby birds (kids) to feed? Here's a dish my son James would surely recommend for a speedy but satisfying supper! If you're cooking for a crowd, this recipe is an easy one to double or triple. James usually likes to live on "the spicier side of the street," but I adjusted the seasoning here for the rest of us.   ☻   Serves 4 (1¼ cups)

8 ounces ground 90% lean turkey or beef
¼ cup chopped onion
10 ounces (one 16-ounce can) pinto beans, rinsed and drained
1¾ cups (one 14½-ounce can) stewed tomatoes, undrained
1 cup (one 8-ounce can) Hunt's Tomato Sauce
1 tablespoon taco seasoning

In a large saucepan sprayed with olive oil–flavored cooking spray, brown meat and onion. Stir in pinto beans, undrained stewed tomatoes, tomato sauce, and taco seasoning. Mix well to combine. Lower heat and simmer for 10 minutes, stirring occasionally.

HINT: For those who like to live on the hotter side of the street, add canned green chili peppers and/or more taco seasoning.

Each serving equals:

HE: 2¾ Protein • 2 Vegetable

225 Calories • 5 gm Fat • 17 gm Protein •
28 gm Carbohydrate • 770 mg Sodium •
91 mg Calcium • 8 gm Fiber

DIABETIC: 2 Meat • 2 Vegetable • 1 Starch

Heartland Corn Chowder

Because Iowa is known for the corn and hogs we raise, and as this rib-sticking combination highlights both corn and lean ham, I just had to name it after the "heartland" of the nation. It's so thick and yummy, you almost need a fork to eat it, and once you've tried it, you'll feel like an honorary Iowan!   ☺   Serves 4 (1¼ cups)

½ cup finely chopped onion
1 full cup (6 ounces) diced Dubuque 97% fat-free ham or any
    extra-lean ham
2 cups frozen whole-kernel corn
1½ cups (8 ounces) diced cooked potatoes
½ cup (one 2.5-ounce jar) sliced mushrooms, drained
1 (10¾-ounce) can Healthy Request Cream of Mushroom Soup
1⅓ cups skim milk
¾ cup (3 ounces) shredded Kraft reduced-fat Cheddar cheese
1 teaspoon prepared mustard
1 teaspoon Sugar Twin or Sprinkle Sweet
1 teaspoon dried parsley flakes
¼ teaspoon black pepper

In a large saucepan sprayed with butter-flavored cooking spray, sauté onion and ham for about 10 minutes or until onion is tender, stirring often. Add corn, potatoes, mushrooms, mushroom soup, and skim milk. Mix well to combine. Stir in Cheddar cheese, mustard, Sugar Twin, parsley flakes, and black pepper. Lower heat and simmer for 10 minutes, stirring occasionally.

Each serving equals:

HE: 2 Protein • 1½ Bread • ½ Vegetable •
⅓ Skim Milk • ½ Slider • 2 Optional Calories

303 Calories • 7 gm Fat • 20 gm Protein •
40 gm Carbohydrate • 973 mg Sodium •
317 mg Calcium • 4 gm Fiber

DIABETIC: 2½ Starch • 2 Meat

New Orleans Bean Soup

They call this Southern home of jazz the Big Easy—and this fast and fabulous recipe serves us a pot of soup that's both really big and oh-so-easy! As they say in Louisiana, let the good times roll!

○ Serves 4 (1½ cups)

½ cup chopped onion

½ cup chopped celery

½ cup shredded carrots

1 full cup (6 ounces) chopped Dubuque 97% fat-free ham or any extra-lean ham

1 teaspoon dried minced garlic

10 ounces (one 16-ounce can) red kidney beans, rinsed and drained

2 cups (one 16-ounce can) Healthy Request Chicken Broth

2 cups water

1 teaspoon Worcestershire sauce

2 tablespoons chopped fresh parsley or 2 teaspoons dried parsley flakes

1 to 2 drops Tabasco sauce

2 teaspoons lemon juice

¼ teaspoon black pepper

In a large saucepan sprayed with butter-flavored cooking spray, sauté onion, celery, and carrots for 5 minutes or until tender. Add ham, garlic, kidney beans, chicken broth, and water. Mix well to combine. Bring mixture to a boil. Stir in Worcestershire sauce, parsley, Tabasco sauce, lemon juice, and black pepper. Lower heat and simmer for 15 minutes, stirring occasionally.

Each serving equals:

HE: 2¼ Protein • ¾ Vegetable • 8 Optional Calories

192 Calories • 4 gm Fat • 21 gm Protein •
18 gm Carbohydrate • 815 mg Sodium •
51 mg Calcium • 6 gm Fiber

DIABETIC: 2 Meat • 1 Starch • 1 Vegetable

Newfoundland Soup

Tasting regional specialties is one of the true pleasures of feasting at our nation's table as I tour to promote my cookbooks. Here's an unusual combination of ingredients that produces a special favorite in Eastern Canada. I bet that no matter where you live, you'll like it! ❤ Serves 4 (1½ cups)

> 2 (2.5-ounce) packages Carl Buddig 90% lean corned beef, shredded
> 2 cups (10 ounces) diced raw potatoes
> 1 cup diced turnips
> 1 cup diced carrots
> ½ cup chopped onion
> 2½ cups water
> 2 cups (one 16-ounce can) tomatoes, coarsely chopped and undrained
> ⅓ cup (1 ounce) uncooked Minute Rice

In a large saucepan, combine corned beef, potatoes, turnips, carrots, onion, and water. Bring mixture to a boil. Stir in undrained tomatoes and uncooked rice. Lower heat, cover, and simmer for 30 to 40 minutes or until vegetables are tender. Stir well just before serving.

HINT: This is a very thick and hearty soup, almost like a stew.

Each serving equals:

HE: 2¼ Vegetable • 1¼ Protein • ¾ Bread

159 Calories • 3 gm Fat • 10 gm Protein •
23 gm Carbohydrate • 531 mg Sodium •
36 mg Calcium • 4 gm Fiber

DIABETIC: 2 Vegetable • 1 Meat • 1 Starch

Savory Salads

Fresh Veggie Salad

What a glory a vegetable garden can be, if you've got the room and the time to cultivate it. But even for those of you who don't, here's a recipe that combines a garden's worth of vegetables into a flavorful dish the whole family will relish. And think of how much stress you can dissolve by chopping, chopping, chopping. . . .

○ Serves 6 (¾ cup)

2 cups chopped fresh cauliflower
2 cups chopped fresh broccoli
1 cup chopped unpeeled cucumber
¾ cup chopped fresh mushrooms
¼ cup sliced green onion
½ cup Kraft fat-free mayonnaise
¼ cup Land O Lakes no-fat sour cream
2 tablespoons Kraft Fat-Free French Dressing
2 teaspoons white vinegar
Sugar substitute to equal 2 teaspoons sugar
¼ teaspoon black pepper

In a large bowl, combine cauliflower, broccoli, cucumber, mushrooms, and green onion. In a small bowl, combine mayonnaise, sour cream, French dressing, vinegar, sugar substitute, and black pepper. Add dressing mixture to vegetable mixture. Mix gently to combine. Cover and refrigerate for at least 1 hour. Gently stir again just before serving.

Each serving equals:

HE: 2 Vegetable • ¼ Slider • 12 Optional Calories

56 Calories • 0 gm Fat • 2 gm Protein •
12 gm Carbohydrate • 256 mg Sodium •
37 mg Calcium • 2 gm Fiber

DIABETIC: 2 Vegetable

Creamy Calico Catalina Veggie Salad

The more colors on the plate, the more anticipation in your mouth, especially when your veggie salad features a creamy combination dressing that says "Party time" with every bite! Even if you can't hop the ferry to this California isle, you can celebrate the flavors it inspired. ☻ Serves 6 (⅔ cup)

¼ cup Kraft Fat-Free Catalina Dressing
¼ cup Kraft Fat-Free Ranch Dressing
1 teaspoon dried parsley flakes
2 cups (one 16-ounce can) whole-kernel corn, rinsed and drained
2 cups (one 16-ounce can) sliced carrots, rinsed and drained
2 cups (one 16-ounce can) cut green beans, rinsed and drained

In a large bowl, combine Catalina dressing, Ranch dressing, and parsley flakes. Add corn, carrots, and green beans. Mix gently to combine. Cover and refrigerate for at least 30 minutes. Gently stir again just before serving.

Each serving equals:

HE: 1⅓ Vegetable • ⅔ Bread • ¼ Slider •
13 Optional Calories

96 Calories • 0 gm Fat • 2 gm Protein •
22 gm Carbohydrate • 244 mg Sodium •
26 mg Calcium • 3 gm Fiber

DIABETIC: 1 Vegetable • 1 Starch

Broccoli-Apple Salad

This unusual combination of sweet, crunchy, and tangy, too, provides lots of "good-for-you" vitamins and not a lot of calories. If one of your goals is increasing the fiber in your diet, put this on your menu as often as you like.   ☯   Serves 6 (⅔ cup)

3 cups chopped fresh broccoli
1½ cups (3 small) cored, unpeeled, and diced Red Delicious
    apples
6 tablespoons raisins
2 tablespoons Hormel Bacon Bits
⅓ cup (1½ ounces) shredded Kraft reduced-fat Cheddar cheese
⅔ cup Kraft fat-free mayonnaise
Sugar substitute to equal 2 tablespoons sugar
1 teaspoon lemon juice

In a large bowl, combine broccoli, apples, raisins, bacon bits, and Cheddar cheese. In a small bowl, combine mayonnaise, sugar substitute, and lemon juice. Add dressing mixture to broccoli mixture. Mix gently to combine. Cover and refrigerate for at least 1 hour. Gently stir again just before serving.

HINT: To plump up raisins without "cooking," place in a glass measuring cup and microwave on HIGH for 30 seconds.

Each serving equals:

HE: 1 Vegetable • 1 Fruit • ⅓ Protein • ¼ Slider •
8 Optional Calories

---

106 Calories • 2 gm Fat • 4 gm Protein •
18 gm Carbohydrate • 382 mg Sodium •
72 mg Calcium • 2 gm Fiber

DIABETIC: 1 Vegetable • 1 Fruit • ½ Fat

French Celery Cabbage Salad

Munch, munch, munch—it's just so satisfying to crunch away on a lively salad like this one! And isn't it great that we can now buy already shredded cabbage in our markets to make speedy preparation even quicker?   ☻   Serves 6 (¾ cup)

3 cups shredded cabbage
1¼ cups chopped celery
¼ cup finely chopped green bell pepper
¼ cup finely chopped onion
¼ cup (one 2-ounce jar) diced pimiento, drained
½ cup Kraft Fat-Free French Dressing
¼ teaspoon black pepper

In a large bowl, combine cabbage, celery, green pepper, onion, and pimiento. Add French dressing and black pepper. Mix well to combine. Cover and refrigerate for at least 1 hour. Gently stir again just before serving.

Each serving equals:

HE: 1⅔ Vegetable • ½ Slider

52 Calories • 0 gm Fat • 1 gm Protein •
12 gm Carbohydrate • 229 mg Sodium •
29 mg Calcium • 1 gm Fiber

DIABETIC: 2 Vegetable *or* 1 Vegetable •
½ Starch/Carbohydrate

Grandma's Cucumbers

Ever stare for a few minutes at the supermarket spice rack and wonder what all those intriguing bottles can do for your food? Since I love to experiment with unfamiliar flavors, I've bought plenty of those bottles and sprinkled them on lots of dishes. Here's one salad that benefits beautifully from a sprinkle of celery seed and lemon pepper.   ☻   Serves 4 (1 scant cup)

> 3 cups thinly sliced unpeeled cucumbers
> ½ cup thinly sliced onion
> Sugar substitute to equal ¼ cup sugar
> ¼ cup white vinegar
> ½ teaspoon celery seed
> ¼ teaspoon lemon pepper

In a medium bowl, combine cucumbers and onion. In a small bowl, combine sugar substitute, vinegar, celery seed, and lemon pepper. Add dressing mixture to cucumber mixture. Mix gently to combine. Cover and refrigerate for at least 1 hour. Gently stir again just before serving.

Each serving equals:

HE: 1¾ Vegetable • 6 Optional Calories

20 Calories • 0 gm Fat • 1 gm Protein •
4 gm Carbohydrate • 3 mg Sodium • 20 mg Calcium •
1 gm Fiber

DIABETIC: 1 Free Vegetable

Carrot Picnic Salad

Take-along food for all those fun family outings seems even more delicious when it's served on paper plates by a sun-dappled lake. This fresh take on carrot salad is sweet and tangy, delivering lots of vitamin A.   ☉   Serves 6 (⅔ cup)

4 cups (two 16-ounce cans) sliced carrots, rinsed and drained
1¼ cups sliced green bell pepper
¾ cup sliced onion
1 (10¾-ounce) can Healthy Request Tomato Soup
½ cup Sugar Twin or Sprinkle Sweet
⅓ cup white vinegar
1 teaspoon dried parsley flakes
¼ teaspoon black pepper

In a large bowl, arrange carrots, green pepper, and onion in layers. In a medium saucepan, combine tomato soup, sugar substitute, vinegar, parsley flakes, and black pepper. Cook over medium heat until mixture just starts to boil, stirring often. Pour hot mixture evenly over vegetables. Mix well to coat vegetables. Cover and refrigerate for at least 2 hours. Gently stir again just before serving.

Each serving equals:

HE: 2 Vegetable • ¼ Slider • 18 Optional Calories

73 Calories • 1 gm Fat • 1 gm Protein •
15 gm Carbohydrate • 196 mg Sodium •
38 mg Calcium • 2 gm Fiber

DIABETIC: 2 Vegetable

Mediterranean Carrot Salad

Here's a new approach to this old favorite—one that is more tangy and less sweet. I think you'll agree it makes a wonderful accompaniment to hearty main dishes and barbecued meats.

◐ Serves 4 (⅔ cup)

> 2½ cups shredded carrots
> 1 cup hot water
> ½ teaspoon dried minced garlic
> 2 tablespoons Kraft Fat-Free Italian Dressing
> ¼ cup Kraft Fat-Free French Dressing
> ½ cup finely chopped green bell pepper

In a medium saucepan, combine carrots, hot water, and garlic. Cook over medium heat for 6 to 8 minutes or until carrots are just tender. Drain well. In a medium bowl, combine Italian dressing and French dressing. Add carrots and green pepper. Mix well to combine. Cover and refrigerate for at least 30 minutes. Gently stir again just before serving.

Each serving equals:

HE: 1½ Vegetable • ¼ Slider • 9 Optional Calories

60 Calories • 0 gm Fat • 1 gm Protein •
14 gm Carbohydrate • 252 mg Sodium •
20 mg Calcium • 2 gm Fiber

DIABETIC: 1 Vegetable • ½ Starch/Carbohydrate

Harvest Carrot Salad

Most traditional carrot salads call for raisins, but I always want more flavors and fruit with mine! By stirring in some apricots and pecans, I've created a dish I think is worthy of serving at a homecoming celebration or anniversary party. ☻ Serves 6 (⅔ cup)

2½ *cups shredded carrots*

½ *cup chopped celery*

2 *cups (one 16-ounce can) apricot halves, packed in fruit juice,*
  drained and coarsely chopped, and 2 tablespoons liquid
  reserved

¼ *cup raisins*

3 *tablespoons (¾ ounce) chopped pecans*

½ *cup Kraft fat-free mayonnaise*

½ *teaspoon apple pie spice*

In a large bowl, combine carrots, celery, apricots, raisins, and pecans. In a small bowl, combine mayonnaise, reserved apricot liquid, and apple pie spice. Add dressing mixture to carrot mixture. Mix well to combine. Cover and refrigerate for at least 1 hour. Gently stir again just before serving.

HINT: To plump up raisins without "cooking," place in a glass measuring cup and microwave on HIGH for 15 seconds.

Each serving equals:

HE: 1 Vegetable • 1 Fruit • ½ Fat •
13 Optional Calories

118 Calories • 2 gm Fat • 1 gm Protein •
24 gm Carbohydrate • 202 mg Sodium •
31 mg Calcium • 3 gm Fiber

DIABETIC: 1 Vegetable • 1 Fruit • ½ Fat

Asparagus-Corn Salad

I just love the yellow and green all stirred up together in this pretty and flavorful special salad. The dressing is sure to provide your taste buds with a wonderful wake-up call! ☻   Serves 6 (½ cup)

1½ cups frozen whole-kernel corn, thawed
2 cups cut fresh or frozen asparagus, cooked and cooled
½ cup Kraft fat-free mayonnaise
1 teaspoon lemon juice
½ teaspoon prepared horseradish sauce
⅛ teaspoon black pepper

In a medium bowl, combine corn and asparagus. In a small bowl, combine mayonnaise, lemon juice, horseradish sauce, and black pepper. Add dressing mixture to corn mixture. Mix gently to combine. Cover and refrigerate for at least 30 minutes. Gently stir again just before serving.

HINT: Thaw corn by placing in a colander and rinsing under hot water for one minute.

Each serving equals:

HE: ¾ Vegetable • ½ Bread • 14 Optional Calories

64 Calories • 0 gm Fat • 2 gm Protein • 14 gm Carbohydrate • 178 mg Sodium • 11 mg Calcium • 2 gm Fiber

DIABETIC: 1 Starch • ½ Vegetable

Inn of the Six-Toed Cat Pea Salad

Isn't this a delightful name for a recipe—and for a place to visit? (It's inspired by a salad I tasted while visiting radio host Bob Finley's bed-and-breakfast inn in Allerton, Iowa.) This pea and rice salad is spiced with some delicate Far Eastern flavors, for a combination that's both original and very hard to resist. So don't resist—eat up!

☙ Serves 6 (½ cup)

½ cup Kraft fat-free mayonnaise
¾ teaspoon curry powder
½ teaspoon turmeric
½ teaspoon ground ginger
2 tablespoons skim milk
1½ cups cold cooked rice
1½ cups frozen peas, thawed
¾ cup finely chopped celery
¼ cup finely chopped onion

In a medium bowl, combine mayonnaise, curry powder, turmeric, ginger, and skim milk. Stir in rice. Let set for 5 minutes. Add peas, celery, and onion. Mix well to combine. Cover and refrigerate for at least 1 hour. Gently stir again just before serving.

HINTS: 1. 1 cup uncooked rice usually cooks to about 1½ cups.
2. Thaw peas by placing in a colander and rinsing under hot water for one minute.

Each serving equals:

HE: 1 Bread • ⅓ Vegetable • 15 Optional Calories

88 Calories • 0 gm Fat • 3 gm Protein •
19 gm Carbohydrate • 192 mg Sodium •
27 mg Calcium • 2 gm Fiber

DIABETIC: 1 Starch

Garden Walnut Salad

It's like finding buried treasure where you never expected when you bite into a bit of walnut in this splendid salad! And you'll think you're getting so much more than one-quarter ounce of nuts per serving. Isn't it great not to feel deprived anymore?

☻ Serves 4 (1¼ cups)

> 3 cups finely shredded lettuce
> ½ cup shredded carrots
> ½ cup thinly sliced unpeeled cucumbers
> ¼ cup (1 ounce) chopped walnuts
> ¼ cup Kraft Fat-Free Ranch Dressing
> 2 tablespoons Kraft Fat-Free Italian Dressing

In a large bowl, combine lettuce, carrots, cucumbers, and walnuts. Refrigerate for at least 30 minutes. Just before serving, combine Ranch and Italian dressings. Add dressing mixture to lettuce mixture. Toss gently to coat. Serve at once.

Each serving equals:

HE: 2 Vegetable • ½ Fat • ¼ Protein • ¼ Slider • 9 Optional Calories

93 Calories • 5 gm Fat • 2 gm Protein • 10 gm Carbohydrate • 247 mg Sodium • 21 mg Calcium • 1 gm Fiber

DIABETIC: 2 Vegetable • 1 Fat

Layered Spinach Salad

Popeye isn't the only person to cheer the health benefits of that dark-green and oh-so-nutritious veggie, spinach, but he's probably the best-known! This is a great way to serve spinach to anyone who isn't sure he likes it . . . and I'll just bet you'll win him over.

☻ Serves 4 (1½ cups)

> 4 cups fresh, torn spinach leaves, stems removed and discarded
> 1¼ cups sliced unpeeled cucumbers
> ½ cup sliced radishes
> ¼ cup sliced green onion
> 2 hard-boiled eggs, sliced
> ½ cup Kraft Fat-Free Ranch Dressing
> ¼ cup Kraft fat-free mayonnaise

Evenly layer spinach, cucumbers, radishes, onion, and eggs in an 8-by-8-inch dish. In a small bowl, combine Ranch dressing and mayonnaise. Spread dressing mixture over top. Cover and refrigerate for at least 2 hours or up to 24 hours. Toss gently just before serving.

Each serving equals:

HE: 3 Vegetable • ½ Protein (limited) • ¾ Slider

115 Calories • 3 gm Fat • 5 gm Protein • 17 gm Carbohydrate • 480 mg Sodium • 77 mg Calcium • 2 gm Fiber

DIABETIC: 2 Vegetable • ½ Meat • ½ Starch/Carbohydrate

Dad's Potato Salad

Couldn't you just gobble down potato salad every day during June, July, and August? (Actually, Cliff could gobble potato salad just about every day of the year!) What's great about this recipe is how much true flavor it imparts, even though I've whisked out most of the fat. ☻ Serves 6 (¾ cup)

3 full cups (16 ounces) diced cooked potatoes
½ cup diced onion
½ cup finely diced celery
¼ cup diced radishes
¼ cup diced green bell pepper
¼ cup Kraft Fat-Free Western Dressing
¼ cup Kraft fat-free mayonnaise
⅛ teaspoon black pepper
2 hard-boiled eggs, diced

In a large bowl, combine potatoes, onion, celery, radishes, and green pepper. In a small bowl, combine Western dressing, mayonnaise, and black pepper. Add dressing mixture to potato mixture. Mix gently to combine. Fold in eggs. Cover and refrigerate for at least 30 minutes. Gently stir again just before serving.

HINT: If you want the look and feel of egg without the cholesterol, toss out the yolks and dice the whites.

Each serving equals:

HE: ⅔ Bread • ½ Vegetable • ⅓ Protein (limited) • ¼ Slider • 3 Optional Calories

---

122 Calories • 2 gm Fat • 3 gm Protein •
23 gm Carbohydrate • 221 mg Sodium •
20 mg Calcium • 2 gm Fiber

DIABETIC: 1½ Starch

Sweet Potato Salad

I love sweet potatoes plain; they're so sweet and rich all on their own! But when I decided to stir them up into this surprising blended salad, I made something already splendid into something sensational! And yes, try it with the pecans sometime for a change of pace. For just a few more calories, you'll feel like you're feasting.

☺ Serves 4 (full ½ cup)

2½ cups (12 ounces) diced cooked sweet potatoes
1 cup diced celery
2 tablespoons Hormel Bacon Bits
¼ cup Kraft Fat-Free Catalina Dressing
2 tablespoons Kraft fat-free mayonnaise
1 teaspoon dried parsley flakes

In a medium bowl, combine sweet potatoes, celery, and bacon bits. In a small bowl, combine Catalina dressing, mayonnaise, and parsley flakes. Add dressing mixture to sweet potato mixture. Mix gently to combine. Cover and refrigerate for at least 1 hour. Gently stir again just before serving.

HINT: Also excellent with 2 tablespoons of chopped pecans stirred in.

Each serving equals:

HE: 1 Bread • ½ Vegetable • ½ Slider •
3 Optional Calories

121 Calories • 1 gm Fat • 3 gm Protein •
25 gm Carbohydrate • 432 mg Sodium •
32 mg Calcium • 3 gm Fiber

DIABETIC: 1½ Starch

Easy Corn Relish

Here's another classic Iowa side dish you may have left off your menu for a while because the traditional recipe was too high in calories and fat. But now you can hop back on the hay wagon and charm your guests with this healthy and tasty version! (It reminds me of my mom's, but it requires much less work.)

○ Serves 8 (¼ cup)

> ¼ cup finely diced green bell pepper
>
> ¼ cup (one 2-ounce jar) chopped pimiento, drained
>
> 2 tablespoons finely chopped onion
>
> ½ cup finely chopped celery
>
> 2 cups (one 16-ounce can) whole-kernel corn, rinsed and drained
>
> ⅓ cup Kraft Fat-Free French Dressing
>
> 1 tablespoon white vinegar

In a medium bowl, combine green pepper, pimiento, onion, celery, and corn. Add French dressing and vinegar. Mix well to combine. Cover and refrigerate for at least 2 hours. Gently stir again just before serving.

Each serving equals:

> HE: ½ Bread • ¼ Vegetable • 17 Optional Calories
>
> ---
>
> 56 Calories • 0 gm Fat • 1 gm Protein •
> 13 gm Carbohydrate • 108 mg Sodium •
> 5 mg Calcium • 1 gm Fiber
>
> ---
>
> DIABETIC: 1 Starch

Mexicalli Pasta Salad

Fiber-rich meals contribute so much to a healthy lifestyle, but many people believe that high-fiber meals can't also be tasty. This slightly spicy side dish I created in response to a reader's request delivers so much flavor and fiber "bang" for the calorie "buck," you'll want to serve it all the time. ☻ Serves 4 (¾ cup)

> 1½ cups cold cooked rotini pasta, rinsed and drained
> 10 ounces (one 16-ounce can) red kidney beans, rinsed and
>   drained
> ⅓ cup Kraft Fat-Free French Dressing
> 1½ teaspoons chili seasoning
> 1 teaspoon dried parsley flakes

In a medium bowl, combine rotini pasta and kidney beans. Add French dressing, chili seasoning, and parsley flakes. Mix well to combine. Cover and refrigerate for at least 1 hour. Gently stir again just before serving.

HINT: 1 full cup uncooked rotini pasta usually cooks to about 1½ cups.

Each serving equals:

HE: 1¼ Protein • ¾ Bread • ¼ Slider • 13 Optional Calories

---

160 Calories • 0 gm Fat • 6 gm Protein • 34 gm Carbohydrate • 200 mg Sodium • 22 mg Calcium • 5 gm Fiber

---

DIABETIC: 2 Starch • 1 Meat

Macaroni, Pea, and Cheese Salad

It seems as if every church and community cookbook features half a dozen macaroni salads, and I think I know why: it's such a wonderfully old-fashioned comfort food, and yet each new way of serving it makes it seem fresh. Try out this combo at your next barbecue, and see if your serving bowl isn't scraped clean!

◑ Serves 6 (¾ cup)

> 2 cups cold cooked rotini pasta, rinsed and drained
> 1 cup frozen peas, thawed
> 1 cup chopped celery
> 2 tablespoons finely chopped onion or 1 teaspoon dried onion
> flakes
> ¾ cup (3 ounces) shredded Kraft reduced-fat Cheddar cheese
> ½ cup Kraft fat-free mayonnaise
> 1 tablespoon Heinz Light Harvest Ketchup or any reduced-sodium
> ketchup
> 1 teaspoon prepared mustard
> 2 tablespoons skim milk
> Sugar substitute to equal 2 teaspoons sugar

In a large bowl, combine rotini pasta, peas, celery, onion, and Cheddar cheese. In a small bowl, combine mayonnaise, ketchup, mustard, skim milk, and sugar substitute. Add dressing mixture to pasta mixture. Mix well to combine. Cover and refrigerate for at least 1 hour. Gently stir again just before serving.

HINTS: 1. 1½ cups uncooked rotini pasta usually cooks to about 2 cups.
2. Thaw peas by placing in a colander and rinsing under hot water for one minute.

Each serving equals:

HE: 1 Bread • ⅔ Protein • ⅓ Vegetable •
18 Optional Calories

147 Calories • 3 gm Fat • 8 gm Protein •
22 gm Carbohydrate • 337 mg Sodium •
127 mg Calcium • 2 gm Fiber

DIABETIC: 1½ Starch • ½ Meat

Layered Lettuce and Ham Salad

If you've never made a layered salad, this one is a great place to start! I've blended some favorite flavors in a fresh way to create a side dish that truly deserves a featured spot on your dinner plate! It also packs a wonderful calcium punch. ☻ Serves 4 (1½ cups)

> 4 cups finely shredded lettuce
> ½ cup chopped onion
> 1 full cup (6 ounces) diced Dubuque 97% fat-free ham or any
>   extra-lean ham
> ¾ cup (3 ounces) shredded Kraft reduced-fat Cheddar cheese
> ¾ cup Yoplait plain fat-free yogurt
> ⅓ cup Carnation Nonfat Dry Milk Powder
> ⅓ cup Kraft fat-free mayonnaise
> Sugar substitute to equal 1 tablespoon sugar
> 1 teaspoon lemon juice
> 1 teaspoon dried parsley flakes

Place lettuce in a 9-by-9-inch cake pan. Layer onion and ham evenly over lettuce. Sprinkle Cheddar cheese over ham. In a small bowl, combine yogurt and dry milk powder. Stir in mayonnaise, sugar substitute, lemon juice, and parsley flakes. Evenly spread dressing mixture over top. Cover and refrigerate for at least 2 hours or up to 24 hours. Toss gently just before serving.

Each serving equals:

HE: 2¼ Vegetable • 2 Protein • ½ Skim Milk •
15 Optional Calories

---

169 Calories • 5 gm Fat • 18 gm Protein •
13 gm Carbohydrate • 754 mg Sodium •
323 mg Calcium • 1 gm Fiber

DIABETIC: 2 Meat • 1 Vegetable •
½ Skim Milk *or* 2 Meat • 1 Starch/Carbohydrate

Ham Salad Combo

Yummy! After just one bite of this delectable salad, that's the unanimous reaction I got when everybody tasted this dish. Make sure you leave enough time for the flavors to join hands and circle round in your refrigerator before you serve it!

○ Serves 4 (1 cup)

> 1½ cups (9 ounces) finely diced Dubuque 97% fat-free ham or any extra-lean ham
> ¾ cup (3 ounces) shredded Kraft reduced-fat Cheddar cheese
> 2 cups (one 16-ounce can) peas, rinsed and drained
> ¼ cup Kraft Fat-Free Thousand Island Dressing
> 2 tablespoons Kraft fat-free mayonnaise

In a medium bowl, combine ham, Cheddar cheese, and peas. Add Thousand Island dressing and mayonnaise. Mix gently to combine. Cover and refrigerate for at least 30 minutes. Gently stir again just before serving.

Each serving equals:

HE: 2½ Protein • 1 Bread • ¼ Slider • 10 Optional Calories

---

206 Calories • 6 gm Fat • 20 gm Protein • 18 gm Carbohydrate • 942 mg Sodium • 170 mg Calcium • 3 gm Fiber

---

DIABETIC: 2 Meat • 1 Starch

Summer Ham and Tomato Pasta Salad

A carnival, with all its wonderful colors and aromas, comes to mind when I contemplate this fresh blended salad! What a great choice for a summer luncheon party, or just an easy way to show your family you think they're special. ☻   Serves 4 (1 full cup)

> 2 cups chopped unpeeled fresh tomatoes
> 1 full cup (6 ounces) diced Dubuque 97% fat-free ham or any
>   extra-lean ham
> ⅓ cup (1½ ounces) shredded Kraft reduced-fat Cheddar cheese
> ¼ cup chopped red onion
> ¼ cup chopped green bell pepper
> 2 cups cold cooked rotini pasta, rinsed and drained
> ¼ cup Kraft Fat-Free Ranch Dressing
> ¼ cup Kraft Fat-Free Catalina Dressing
> 1 tablespoon chopped fresh parsley or 1 teaspoon dried parsley
>   flakes

In a large bowl, combine tomatoes, ham, Cheddar cheese, onion, and green pepper. Stir in rotini pasta. In a small bowl, combine Ranch dressing, Catalina dressing, and parsley. Add dressing mixture to pasta mixture. Mix gently to combine. Cover and refrigerate for at least 1 hour. Gently stir again just before serving.

HINT: 1½ cups uncooked rotini pasta usually cooks to about 2 cups.

Each serving equals:

> HE: 1½ Protein • 1¼ Vegetable • 1 Bread •
> ½ Slider • 10 Optional Calories
>
> ---
>
> 236 Calories • 4 gm Fat • 14 gm Protein •
> 36 gm Carbohydrate • 786 mg Sodium •
> 81 mg Calcium • 2 gm Fiber
>
> ---
>
> DIABETIC: 2 Starch • 1½ Meat • 1 Vegetable

Lazy Dog Macaroni Salad

Even the sleepiest pup would hop up and run over when you're dishing out this quick-to-fix festive salad! You'll surely be "top dog" at your house any time you put this on the menu.

○ Serves 4 (⅔ cup)

> 1½ cups cold cooked elbow macaroni, rinsed and drained
> ½ cup frozen peas, thawed
> ¾ cup (3 ounces) shredded Kraft reduced-fat Cheddar cheese
> ¼ cup Kraft fat-free mayonnaise
> ¼ cup sweet pickle relish
> 1 teaspoon dried onion flakes
> ¼ teaspoon black pepper

In a large bowl, combine macaroni, peas, and Cheddar cheese. In a small bowl, combine mayonnaise, pickle relish, onion flakes, and black pepper. Add dressing mixture to macaroni mixture. Mix well to combine. Cover and refrigerate for at least 30 minutes. Gently stir again just before serving.

HINTS: 1. 1 full cup uncooked elbow macaroni usually cooks to about 1½ cups.
2. Thaw peas by placing in a colander and rinsing under hot water for one minute.

Each serving equals:

HE: 1 Bread • 1 Protein • ¼ Slider •
5 Optional Calories

---

180 Calories • 4 gm Fat • 10 gm Protein •
26 gm Carbohydrate • 436 mg Sodium •
166 mg Calcium • 2 gm Fiber

DIABETIC: 1½ Starch • 1 Meat

Reuben Pasta Salad

In its original version, the Reuben sandwich is so full of fat and calories, a health-conscious eater wouldn't dare order one at a favorite deli restaurant! But here's a salad that provides the tastes you simply adore, with most of the fat and calories whisked out with Healthy Exchanges magic. Try this on St. Paddy's Day—or any time at all!   ☻   Serves 4 (1 full cup)

> 2 cups cold cooked rotini pasta, rinsed and drained
> 2 (2.5-ounce) packages Carl Buddig 90% lean corned beef, shredded
> 3 (¾-ounce) slices Kraft reduced-fat Swiss cheese, shredded
> ¼ cup finely chopped onion
> 1¾ cups (one 14½-ounce can) Frank's Bavarian-style sauerkraut, drained
> ¼ cup Kraft Fat-Free Thousand Island Dressing
> 2 tablespoons Kraft fat-free mayonnaise

In a large bowl, combine rotini pasta, corned beef, Swiss cheese, onion, and sauerkraut. In a small bowl, combine Thousand Island dressing and mayonnaise. Add dressing mixture to pasta mixture. Mix gently to combine. Cover and refrigerate for at least 30 minutes. Gently stir again just before serving.

HINTS: 1. 1½ cups uncooked rotini pasta usually cooks to about 2 cups.
2. If you can't find Bavarian-style sauerkraut, use regular sauerkraut, ½ teaspoon caraway seeds, and 1 teaspoon Brown Sugar Twin.

Each serving equals:

HE: 2 Protein • 1 Bread • 1 Vegetable • ¼ Slider • 10 Optional Calories

224 Calories • 4 gm Fat • 16 gm Protein • 31 gm Carbohydrate • 1,403 mg Sodium • 189 mg Calcium • 4 gm Fiber

DIABETIC: 2 Meat • 1½ Starch • 1 Vegetable

Sweet Salads

Fresh Blueberry Kiwi Salad

Fresh blueberries feel like a luxury sometimes, but just like that hair color commercial says, "You're worth it!" Treat yourself and your family to this sweet and tart salad that will make you feel good in every way. ☻ Serves 4 (¾ cup)

> 1 (4-serving) package JELL-O sugar-free instant vanilla pudding mix
> 1 (4-serving) package JELL-O sugar-free lemon gelatin
> ⅔ cup Carnation Nonfat Dry Milk Powder
> 1 cup water
> ¾ cup Yoplait plain fat-free yogurt
> ¼ cup Cool Whip Free
> ¾ cup fresh blueberries
> 1 cup (2 medium) peeled and coarsely chopped kiwi fruit

In a medium bowl, combine dry pudding mix, dry gelatin, and dry milk powder. Add water and yogurt. Mix well using a wire whisk. Blend in Cool Whip Free. Add blueberries and kiwi fruit. Mix gently to combine. Cover and refrigerate for at least 30 minutes. Gently stir again just before serving.

Each serving equals:

HE: ¾ Fruit • ¾ Skim Milk • ½ Slider •
3 Optional Calories

---

140 Calories • 0 gm Fat • 8 gm Protein •
27 gm Carbohydrate • 484 mg Sodium •
234 mg Calcium • 1 gm Fiber

DIABETIC: 1 Fruit • 1 Skim Milk

Heavenly Blueberry Salad

Here's one of my favorite ways to show how partial I am to the red-white-and-blue! Whether you're planning a Flag Day picnic or a barbecue before you all go to the fireworks, why not serve a luscious dish that proudly displays your love for America?

○ Serves 8

1 (4-serving) package JELL-O sugar-free raspberry gelatin
1 cup boiling water
¾ cup Diet Mountain Dew
1 cup (one 8-ounce can) crushed pineapple, packed in fruit, undrained

1½ cups fresh blueberries
¼ cup (1 ounce) chopped pecans
1 (8-ounce) package Philadelphia fat-free cream cheese
1 cup Cool Whip Free
1 teaspoon coconut extract
2 tablespoons flaked coconut

In a large bowl, combine dry gelatin and boiling water. Mix well to dissolve gelatin. Stir in Diet Mountain Dew and undrained pineapple. Pour mixture into an 8-by-8-inch dish. Refrigerate for 30 minutes. Stir in blueberries and pecans. Refrigerate until firm, about 3 hours. In a medium bowl, stir cream cheese with a spoon until soft. Add Cool Whip Free and coconut extract. Mix gently to combine. Evenly spread cream cheese mixture over set gelatin. Sprinkle coconut evenly over top. Refrigerate for at least 30 minutes. Cut into 8 servings.

HINT: Frozen unsweetened blueberries, thawed and drained, may be used in place of fresh.

Each serving equals:

HE: ½ Fruit • ½ Fat • ½ Protein • ¼ Slider • 4 Optional Calories

107 Calories • 3 gm Fat • 5 gm Protein • 15 gm Carbohydrate • 209 mg Sodium • 8 mg Calcium • 1 gm Fiber

DIABETIC: ½ Fruit • ½ Starch/Carbohydrate • ½ Fat • ½ Meat *or* 1 Fruit • ½ Fat • ½ Meat

Crunchy Peach Salad

You know how it feels when you enter a party full of people you don't know and you wonder if you'll find anyone to talk to—but you always do? This salad provides the same sort of appetizing surprise, by inviting the summer's best peaches to shake hands with a few strangers (celery, pecans, maple syrup) who will turn out to be friends!   ☻   Serves 6 (⅔ cup)

> 2 cups (4 medium) peeled and sliced fresh peaches
> 1 cup chopped celery
> ¼ cup raisins
> 3 tablespoons (¾ ounce) chopped pecans
> ¼ cup Kraft fat-free mayonnaise
> ¼ teaspoon ground nutmeg
> 2 tablespoons Cary's Sugar Free Maple Syrup

In a medium bowl, combine peaches, celery, raisins, and pecans. In a small bowl, combine mayonnaise, nutmeg, and maple syrup. Add dressing mixture to peach mixture. Mix gently to combine. Cover and refrigerate for at least 15 minutes. Gently stir again just before serving.

HINT: To plump up raisins without "cooking," place in a glass measuring cup and microwave on HIGH for 15 seconds.

Each serving equals:

HE: 1 Fruit • ½ Fat • ⅓ Vegetable • 10 Optional Calories

82 Calories • 2 gm Fat • 1 gm Protein • 15 gm Carbohydrate • 116 mg Sodium • 15 mg Calcium • 2 gm Fiber

DIABETIC: 1 Fruit • ½ Fat

Creamy Apple–Peanut Butter Salad

This concoction is kind of a Waldorf salad that had a brief but happy encounter with a jar of peanut butter! If your goal is to get your family eating more fruit, slip 'em a spoonful of this festive delight.   ☻   Serves 6 (½ cup)

¾ cup Yoplait plain fat-free yogurt

⅓ cup Carnation Nonfat Dry Milk Powder

¼ cup Peter Pan reduced-fat creamy peanut butter

¼ cup Cool Whip Free

Sugar substitute to equal 2 tablespoons sugar

1 teaspoon vanilla extract

2 cups (4 small) cored, unpeeled, and chopped Red Delicious apples

¼ cup raisins

¾ cup chopped celery

In a large bowl, combine yogurt and dry milk powder. Add peanut butter. Mix well to combine. Stir in Cool Whip Free, sugar substitute, and vanilla extract. Add apples, raisins, and celery. Mix well to combine. Cover and refrigerate for at least 30 minutes. Gently stir again just before serving.

HINT: To plump up raisins without "cooking," place in a glass measuring cup and microwave on HIGH for 15 seconds.

Each serving equals:

HE: 1 Fruit • ⅔ Fat • ⅔ Protein • ⅓ Skim Milk • ¼ Vegetable • 7 Optional Calories

---

135 Calories • 3 gm Fat • 6 gm Protein • 21 gm Carbohydrate • 107 mg Sodium • 114 mg Calcium • 2 gm Fiber

---

DIABETIC: 1 Fruit • ½ Fat • ½ Starch/Carbohydrate

Apple-Scotch Salad

I'm one of those people who enjoys variety on my plate at every meal, so I rarely focus just on a main dish at lunch or dinner. (And my cookbooks reflect this, featuring lots and lots of tasty side dishes!) Give this one a try—it may become the "apple of your eye" as far as salads go. Two of the apples of *my* eye, my daughter-in-law Pam and grandson Zach, both love it.

◐   Serves 8 (½ cup)

> 1 (4-serving) package JELL-O sugar-free instant butterscotch
>   pudding mix
> ⅔ cup Carnation Nonfat Dry Milk Powder
> 1⅓ cups water
> ¼ cup Peter Pan reduced-fat peanut butter
> ⅓ cup Cool Whip Free
> 4 cups (8 small) cored, unpeeled, and diced Red Delicious apples

In a large bowl, combine dry pudding mix and dry milk powder. Add water and peanut butter. Mix well using a wire whisk. Stir in Cool Whip Free. Add apples. Mix well to combine. Cover and refrigerate for at least 30 minutes. Gently stir again just before serving.

Each serving equals:

HE: 1 Fruit • ½ Protein • ½ Fat • ¼ Skim Milk • 18 Optional Calories

119 Calories • 3 gm Fat • 4 gm Protein • 19 gm Carbohydrate • 240 mg Sodium • 73 mg Calcium • 1 gm Fiber

DIABETIC: 1 Fruit • ½ Starch • ½ Fat

Tea Room Apple Salad

This cousin of the Waldorf salad is heartier with the addition of Cheddar cheese and an even creamier dressing than the traditional mix. Turn your kitchen table into a charming setting for afternoon tea, if you like, or just enjoy this recipe when the 4-o'clock munchies "attack" you at work!   ☯   Serves 6 (⅔ cup)

> 1½ cups (3 small) cored, unpeeled, and diced Red Delicious
>   apples
> 1 cup finely chopped celery
> 6 tablespoons raisins
> ¼ cup (1 ounce) chopped walnuts
> ⅓ cup (1½ ounces) shredded Kraft reduced-fat Cheddar cheese
> ⅓ cup Kraft fat-free mayonnaise
> 2 tablespoons Land O Lakes no-fat sour cream
> Lettuce leaves

In a large bowl, combine apples, celery, raisins, walnuts, and Cheddar cheese. In a small bowl, combine mayonnaise and sour cream. Add dressing mixture to apple mixture. Mix gently to combine. Cover and refrigerate for at least 30 minutes. Gently stir again just before serving. Serve on lettuce leaves.

HINT: To plump up raisins without "cooking," place in a glass measuring cup and microwave on HIGH for 30 seconds.

Each serving equals:

> HE: 1 Fruit • ½ Protein • ⅓ Fat • ⅓ Vegetable •
> 14 Optional Calories
> _____
> 112 Calories • 4 gm Fat • 3 gm Protein •
> 16 gm Carbohydrate • 197 mg Sodium •
> 69 mg Calcium • 1 gm Fiber
> _____
> DIABETIC: 1 Fruit • 1 Fat

Dessert Waldorf Salad

I think it was Mae West who was fond of saying, "Too much of a good thing is wonderful!" I bet she'd use those words to describe this pretty dish just overflowing with fruit and other goodies.

○ Serves 8 (½ cup)

> 1 (4-serving) package JELL-O sugar-free instant vanilla pudding
> mix
> ⅔ cup Carnation Nonfat Dry Milk Powder
> 1½ cups water
> ⅓ cup Cool Whip Free
> 1 teaspoon vanilla extract
> 1 cup (2 small) cored, unpeeled, and chopped Red Delicious
> apples
> ¼ cup raisins
> 1 cup (6 ounces) green seedless grapes, halved
> 1 cup (one 8-ounce can) pineapple tidbits, packed in fruit juice,
> drained
> ½ cup (1 ounce) miniature marshmallows
> 2 tablespoons (½ ounce) chopped pecans

In a large bowl, combine dry pudding mix, dry milk powder, and water. Mix well using a wire whisk. Blend in Cool Whip Free and vanilla extract. Add apples, raisins, grapes, pineapple, marshmallows, and pecans. Mix gently to combine. Cover and refrigerate for at least 30 minutes. Gently stir again just before serving.

HINTS: 1. If you can't find pineapple tidbits, use pineapple chunks and coarsely chop.
2. To plump up raisins without "cooking," place in a glass measuring cup and microwave on HIGH for 15 seconds.

Each serving equals:

HE: 1 Fruit • ¼ Skim Milk • ¼ Fat • ¼ Slider • 4 Optional Calories

---

117 Calories • 1 gm Fat • 3 gm Protein • 24 gm Carbohydrate • 200 mg Sodium • 79 mg Calcium • 1 gm Fiber

---

DIABETIC: 1 Fruit • ½ Starch/Carbohydrate

California Apple-Raisin Salad

Here's a fun food fact for you: Fresno, California, is the country's raisin capital. But you don't have to be from that golden state to revel in the glories of this scrumptious combination. It also features the king of nuts, in my humble opinion—mmm, pecans!

◎ Serves 6 (½ cup)

> 1 (4-serving) package JELL-O sugar-free instant vanilla pudding
>   mix
> ⅔ cup Carnation Nonfat Dry Milk Powder
> 1¼ cups water
> 1 teaspoon vanilla extract
> ¼ cup Cool Whip Free
> ½ teaspoon apple pie spice
> 1½ cups (3 small) cored, unpeeled, and diced Red Delicious
>   apples
> 6 tablespoons raisins
> 2 tablespoons (½ ounce) chopped pecans

In a large bowl, combine dry pudding mix, dry milk powder, and water. Mix well using a wire whisk. Blend in vanilla extract, Cool Whip Free, and apple pie spice. Add apples, raisins, and pecans. Mix well to combine. Cover and refrigerate for at least 30 minutes. Gently stir again just before serving.

HINT: To plump up raisins without "cooking," place in a glass measuring cup and microwave on HIGH for 30 seconds.

Each serving equals:

HE: 1 Fruit • ⅓ Fat • ⅓ Skim Milk • ¼ Slider • 2 Optional Calories

---

110 Calories • 2 gm Fat • 3 gm Protein • 20 gm Carbohydrate • 120 mg Sodium • 99 mg Calcium • 1 gm Fiber

---

DIABETIC: 1 Fruit • ½ Starch/Carbohydrate

Judy's Cranberry Salad

This looks just as delicious as the ingredients make it sound! There's something so outrageously good about the combo of cranberries and oranges, you'll want to serve this all year long, not just at the holidays. It's a terrific dish to serve at a graduation party, or perhaps when your in-laws are coming for supper. ☻ Serves 6

1½ cups Ocean Spray reduced-calorie cranberry juice cocktail
1 (4-serving) package JELL-O sugar-free orange gelatin
½ cup unsweetened applesauce
1½ cups fresh or frozen cranberries, coarsely chopped
1 cup (one 11-ounce can) mandarin oranges, rinsed and drained
1 (8-ounce) package Philadelphia fat-free cream cheese
½ cup Cool Whip Free
1 teaspoon vanilla extract
Sugar substitute to equal 2 tablespoons sugar
2 tablespoons (½ ounce) chopped pecans

In a medium saucepan, bring cranberry juice cocktail to a boil. Remove from heat. Stir in dry gelatin. Mix well using a wire whisk to dissolve gelatin. Stir in applesauce. Add cranberries and mandarin oranges. Mix well to combine. Pour mixture into an 8-by-8-inch dish. Refrigerate until firm, about 3 hours. In a medium bowl, stir cream cheese with a spoon until soft. Add Cool Whip Free, vanilla extract, and sugar substitute. Mix well to combine. Spread mixture evenly over set gelatin. Sprinkle pecans evenly over top. Refrigerate for 30 minutes. Cut into 6 servings.

Each serving equals:

HE: 1 Fruit • ⅔ Protein • ⅓ Fat •
19 Optional Calories

114 Calories • 2 gm Fat • 7 gm Protein •
17 gm Carbohydrate • 278 mg Sodium •
8 mg Calcium • 1 gm Fiber

DIABETIC: 1 Fruit • ½ Meat

Mountain Cranberry Holiday Salad

This is a truly yummy accompaniment to your groaning Thanksgiving table, but it's also a delicious way to celebrate any time. Can't you just see this beautifully rosy salad alongside a pale-colored meat like turkey or pork? Mmm-hmm . . .

◐ Serves 8

2 cups fresh or frozen whole cranberries
1 cup Ocean Spray reduced-calorie cranberry juice cocktail
½ cup Sugar Twin or Sprinkle Sweet
1 (4-serving) package JELL-O sugar-free cherry gelatin
1½ cups Diet Mountain Dew ☆
1 cup chopped celery
1½ cups (3 small) cored, unpeeled, and diced Red Delicious apples
¼ cup (1 ounce) chopped pecans ☆
1 (4-serving) package JELL-O sugar-free instant vanilla pudding mix
⅔ cup Carnation Nonfat Dry Milk Powder
½ cup Cool Whip Free
3 to 4 drops red food coloring

In a medium saucepan, combine cranberries, cranberry juice cocktail, and sugar substitute. Cook over medium heat until cranberries become soft, stirring often. Remove from heat. Stir in dry gelatin and ½ cup Diet Mountain Dew. Mix well to dissolve gelatin. Add celery, apples, and 2 tablespoons pecans. Mix well to combine. Pour mixture into an 8-by-8-inch dish. Refrigerate for 2 hours. In a medium bowl, combine dry pudding mix and dry milk powder. Add remaining 1 cup Diet Mountain Dew. Mix well using a wire whisk. Blend in Cool Whip Free and red food coloring. Spread pudding mixture evenly over partially set cranberry mixture. Sprinkle remaining 2 tablespoons pecans over top. Refrigerate for at least 1 hour or until gelatin is firm. Cut into 8 servings.

Each serving equals:

HE: ¾ Fruit • ½ Fat • ¼ Vegetable • ¼ Skim Milk •
¼ Slider • 11 Optional Calories

107 Calories • 3 gm Fat • 3 gm Protein •
17 gm Carbohydrate • 248 mg Sodium •
79 mg Calcium • 2 gm Fiber

DIABETIC: 1 Fruit • ½ Fat

Sharon's Pistachio Salad

Pistachio pudding inspires me to all kinds of fun in the kitchen!
This is a great last-minute dish that looks special and tastes even
better than it looks. It also delivers a nice wallop of calcium in every
serving.   ☻   Serves 4 (1 cup)

> 2 cups (two 8-ounce cans) crushed pineapple, packed in fruit
>   juice, drained
> 1½ cups Yoplait plain fat-free yogurt
> 1 (4-serving) package JELL-O sugar-free instant pistachio pudding
>   mix

In a medium bowl, combine pineapple and yogurt. Add dry
pudding mix. Mix well using a wire whisk. Cover and refrigerate for
at least 30 minutes. Gently stir again just before serving.

Each serving equals:

HE: 1 Fruit • ½ Skim Milk • ¼ Slider •
5 Optional Calories

148 Calories • 0 gm Fat • 5 gm Protein •
32 gm Carbohydrate • 385 mg Sodium •
187 mg Calcium • 1 gm Fiber

DIABETIC: 1 Fruit • 1 Starch/Carbohydrate

Cherry Cola Salad

Oh, remember those golden days of childhood, when you asked the man behind the soda fountain to mix you up the best cherry Coke in town? I do! Now I'm celebrating those good memories, and the flavors you never forgot, in this luscious fruit-and-nutty salad.

○ Serves 8

> 1 cup (one 8-ounce can) crushed pineapple, packed in fruit juice, drained, and ¼ cup liquid reserved
>
> ¾ cup water
>
> 1 (4-serving) package JELL-O sugar-free cherry gelatin
>
> 1 (8-ounce) package Philadelphia fat-free cream cheese
>
> ¾ cup diet Coke
>
> 2 cups (12 ounces) bing cherries, pitted and halved
>
> ¼ cup (1 ounce) chopped pecans

In a small saucepan, combine reserved pineapple liquid and water. Bring mixture to a boil. In a large bowl, combine dry gelatin and boiling liquid. Mix well to dissolve gelatin. Add cream cheese. Mix well using a wire whisk until smooth. Stir in diet Coke. Fold in pineapple, cherries, and pecans. Pour mixture into an 8-by-8-inch dish. Refrigerate until firm, about 3 hours. Cut into 8 servings.

HINT: Bing cherries are also known as dark sweet cherries.

Each serving equals:

> HE: ¾ Fruit • ½ Fat • ½ Protein •
> 5 Optional Calories
>
> ---
> 99 Calories • 3 gm Fat • 5 gm Protein •
> 13 gm Carbohydrate • 198 mg Sodium •
> 12 mg Calcium • 1 gm Fiber
>
> ---
> DIABETIC: 1 Fruit • ½ Fat • ½ Meat

Denise's Spring Dew Salad

One of my newsletter readers, Denise Wagner, said she based this salad on my refreshing and colorful Spring Dew Pie. Serving this is a great way to show your appreciation for the babysitter who makes your life easier, or the neighbor who takes in your packages when you're not home. Isn't there someone in your life you'd like to thank with this sweet treat? ☻ Serves 8

1 cup unsweetened applesauce

1 cup unsweetened orange juice

2 (4-serving) packages JELL-O sugar-free orange gelatin

1 cup Diet Mountain Dew

1 cup (one 8-ounce can) pineapple chunks, packed in fruit juice, drained

1 cup (one 11-ounce can) mandarin oranges, rinsed and drained

In a small saucepan, combine applesauce and orange juice. Bring mixture to a boil. Remove from heat. Add dry gelatin. Mix well to dissolve gelatin. Stir in Diet Mountain Dew. Add pineapple and mandarin oranges. Mix well to combine. Pour mixture into an 8-by-8-inch dish. Refrigerate until firm, about 3 hours. Cut into 8 servings.

Each serving equals:

HE: 1 Fruit • 10 Optional Calories

68 Calories • 0 gm Fat • 2 gm Protein •
15 gm Carbohydrate • 60 mg Sodium •
11 mg Calcium • 1 gm Fiber

DIABETIC: 1 Fruit

Valentine Party Salad

Delicious foods made with a loving heart can be a wonderfully romantic gift to the man you love, especially if you've chosen the ingredients with his good health in mind! This dish should make him smack his lips and, once he's finished, kiss the cook!

○ Serves 6 (⅔ cup)

> 1 (4-serving) package JELL-O sugar-free cherry gelatin
> 2 cups fat-free cottage cheese
> 1 cup (one 8-ounce can) crushed pineapple, packed in fruit juice, drained
> ½ cup (1 ounce) miniature marshmallows
> 2 tablespoons (½ ounce) chopped pecans
> 6 maraschino cherries, quartered
> ¾ cup Cool Whip Free

In a medium bowl, combine dry gelatin and cottage cheese. Fold in pineapple, marshmallows, pecans, and maraschino cherries. Add Cool Whip Free. Mix gently to combine. Cover and refrigerate for at least 30 minutes. Gently stir again just before serving.

Each serving equals:

HE: ⅔ Protein • ⅓ Fat • ⅓ Fruit • ¼ Slider • 13 Optional Calories

138 Calories • 2 gm Fat • 11 gm Protein • 19 gm Carbohydrate • 325 mg Sodium • 39 mg Calcium • 0 gm Fiber

DIABETIC: 1 Meat • 1 Starch/Carbohydrate

Orange Rice Salad

Fruited rice salads are a Midwestern tradition that I hope everyone, everywhere, will decide to try! It's easily digestible, very appealing to both children and adults, and just full of good-for-you goodness.

◐ Serves 6 (⅔ cup)

> *1 cup (one 8-ounce can) pineapple tidbits, packed in fruit juice, undrained*
> *¾ cup Yoplait plain fat-free yogurt*
> *⅓ cup Carnation Nonfat Dry Milk Powder*
> *Sugar substitute to equal 1 tablespoon sugar*
> *1 (4-serving) package JELL-O sugar-free orange gelatin*
> *¾ cup Cool Whip Free*
> *2 cups cold cooked rice*
> *1 cup (one 11-ounce can) mandarin oranges, rinsed and drained*

In a large bowl, combine undrained pineapple, yogurt, dry milk powder, and sugar substitute. Stir in dry gelatin and Cool Whip Free. Add rice and mandarin oranges. Mix gently to combine. Cover and refrigerate for at least 30 minutes. Gently stir again just before serving.

HINTS: 1. 1⅓ cups uncooked rice usually cooks to about 2 cups.
2. If you can't find pineapple tidbits, use pineapple chunks and coarsely chop.

Each serving equals:

HE: ⅔ Bread • ⅔ Fruit • ⅓ Skim Milk • ¼ Slider • 3 Optional Calories

144 Calories • 0 gm Fat • 5 gm Protein • 31 gm Carbohydrate • 87 mg Sodium • 117 mg Calcium • 1 gm Fiber

DIABETIC: 1½ Starch/Carbohydrate • ½ Fruit

Tasty Fruit and Macaroni Salad

Cliff loves macaroni salad, whether it's the traditional savory kind mixed with a tangy dressing and veggies, or the more unusual sort—blended with all kinds of fruit. There's a surprise in every spoonful of this inviting salad, sure to please family members from 2 to 92! ☺ Serves 8 (½ cup)

> 1 cup (one 8-ounce can) pineapple tidbits, packed in fruit juice,
>   drained, and 2 tablespoons liquid reserved
> ¼ cup raisins
> 1 cup (one 11-ounce can) mandarin oranges, rinsed and drained
> 1 cup (2 small) cored, unpeeled, and diced Red Delicious apples
> ½ cup (1 ounce) miniature marshmallows
> ½ cup Kraft fat-free mayonnaise
> Sugar substitute to equal 1 tablespoon sugar
> 2 cups cold cooked elbow macaroni, rinsed and drained

In a large bowl, combine pineapple, raisins, mandarin oranges, apples, and marshmallows. Add mayonnaise, sugar substitute, and reserved pineapple juice. Mix well to combine. Stir in macaroni. Cover and refrigerate for at least 30 minutes. Gently stir again just before serving.

HINTS: 1. If you can't find pineapple tidbits, use pineapple chunks and coarsely chop.
2. To plump up raisins without "cooking," place in a glass measuring cup and microwave on HIGH for 15 seconds.
3. 1⅓ cups uncooked elbow macaroni usually cooks to about 2 cups.

Each serving equals:

HE: 1 Fruit • ½ Bread • 17 Optional Calories

120 Calories • 0 gm Fat • 2 gm Protein •
28 gm Carbohydrate • 134 mg Sodium •
14 mg Calcium • 1 gm Fiber

DIABETIC: 1 Fruit • ½ Starch/Carbohydrate

Vegetables

Aztec Corn Dish

This is a favorite end-of-summer recipe, perfect for when your harvest of zucchini overflows every basket you've got! Brimming with great fresh flavor and color, this is one side dish that doesn't deserve second billing. ☺ Serves 4 (1 full cup)

> 2 cups sliced unpeeled zucchini
> ½ cup chopped onion
> ½ cup chopped green bell pepper
> ½ cup water
> 1½ cups peeled and chopped fresh tomatoes
> 1½ cups frozen whole-kernel corn, thawed
> ¼ teaspoon black pepper
> 1 teaspoon chili seasoning

In a large skillet sprayed with butter-flavored cooking spray, sauté zucchini, onion, and green pepper for 2 to 3 minutes. Add water. Mix well to combine. Cover and cook over medium-high heat for 5 minutes, stirring occasionally. Stir in tomatoes, corn, black pepper, and chili seasoning. Re-cover and continue cooking for 5 to 6 minutes or until vegetables are tender, stirring occasionally.

HINT: Thaw corn by placing in a colander and rinsing under hot water for one minute.

Each serving equals:

HE: 2¼ Vegetable • ¾ Bread

92 Calories • 0 gm Fat • 3 gm Protein • 20 gm Carbohydrate • 12 mg Sodium • 20 mg Calcium • 3 gm Fiber

DIABETIC: 1 Vegetable • 1 Starch

Sweet and Sour Green Beans

Cliff was delighted when I served up this unusual but delicious green bean dish that gives an "everyday" vegetable a little extra zing! Remember to use real bacon bits in this dish, not a soy substitute.

○ Serves 4 (1 scant cup)

½ cup chopped onion
⅓ cup Kraft Fat Free French Dressing
1 tablespoon white vinegar
2 teaspoons Sugar Twin or Sprinkle Sweet
1 teaspoon dried parsley flakes
2 tablespoons Hormel Bacon Bits
4 cups (two 16-ounce cans) French-style green beans, rinsed and
*   drained*

In a large skillet sprayed with butter-flavored cooking spray, sauté onion for 5 minutes or until tender. Stir in French dressing, vinegar, sugar substitute, parsley flakes, and bacon bits. Add green beans. Mix well to combine. Lower heat and simmer for 10 minutes or until mixture is heated through, stirring often.

Each serving equals:

HE: 2¼ Vegetable • ½ Slider • 7 Optional Calories

85 Calories • 1 gm Fat • 3 gm Protein •
16 gm Carbohydrate • 327 mg Sodium •
41 mg Calcium • 2 gm Fiber

DIABETIC: 2 Vegetable • ½ Starch

Mom's Comfort Green Beans

You know how good it feels to go home and have Mom cook all your favorite dishes for you? Well, we don't get to visit our moms as often as we'd like, but recalling those good feelings with every bite of these flavorful green beans brings her close to us in spirit!

◑ Serves 4 (1½ cups)

> 1 full cup (6 ounces) diced Dubuque 97% fat-free ham or any
>   extra-lean ham
> 5 cups frozen or fresh cut green beans
> 3 cups (15 ounces) diced raw potatoes
> ½ cup finely chopped onion
> ¾ cup water
> ¼ teaspoon black pepper
> 2 or 3 drops Tabasco sauce

In a large saucepan sprayed with butter-flavored cooking spray, sauté ham until browned. Add green beans, potatoes, onion, and water. Mix well to combine. Bring mixture to a boil. Stir in black pepper and Tabasco sauce. Continue cooking until beans and potatoes are tender and most of liquid is absorbed.

Each serving equals:

HE: 2¾ Vegetable • 1 Protein • ¾ Bread

116 Calories • 0 gm Fat • 5 gm Protein •
24 gm Carbohydrate • 69 mg Sodium •
55 mg Calcium • 4 gm Fiber

DIABETIC: 2 Vegetable • 1 Meat • 1 Starch

Deviled Green Beans

When I served this dish to Cliff, I spotted a devilish glint of pleasure in his eyes! It tastes wonderfully wicked, but you can eat it as often as you like with a saint's clear conscience!

● Serves 4

2 teaspoons reduced-calorie margarine

1 teaspoon prepared mustard

½ teaspoon Worcestershire sauce

¼ teaspoon black pepper

2 cups (one 16-ounce can) cut green beans, rinsed and drained

½ cup (¾ ounce) crushed cornflakes

In an 8-by-8-inch glass baking dish, combine margarine, mustard, Worcestershire sauce, and black pepper. Microwave on HIGH for 30 seconds. Add green beans. Mix well to combine. Evenly sprinkle cornflakes over top. Microwave on HIGH for 4 to 5 minutes. Let set for 2 to 3 minutes. Divide into 4 servings.

Each serving equals:

HE: 1 Vegetable • ¼ Fat • ¼ Bread

28 Calories • 0 gm Fat • 1 gm Protein •
6 gm Carbohydrate • 66 mg Sodium •
20 mg Calcium • 1 gm Fiber

DIABETIC: 1 Vegetable

Father's Special Green Beans

Any day you serve these creamy, cheesy beans deserves to be called Father's Day, don't you think? Just place a scoop of this tasty dish on his plate, and he'll know instantly that you think he's special!

❂ Serves 6

> 4 cups (two 16-ounce cans) cut green beans, rinsed and drained
> 1 (10¾-ounce) can Healthy Request Cream of Mushroom Soup
> ⅔ cup (2¼ ounces) shredded Kraft reduced-fat Cheddar cheese
> 1 teaspoon dried onion flakes

Preheat oven to 350 degrees. Spray an 8-by-8-inch baking dish with butter-flavored cooking spray. In a large bowl, combine green beans, mushroom soup, Cheddar cheese, and onion flakes. Pour mixture into prepared baking dish. Bake for 30 minutes. Place baking dish on a wire rack and let set for 2 to 3 minutes. Divide into 6 servings.

Each serving equals:

HE: 1⅓ Vegetable • ½ Protein • ¼ Slider • 8 Optional Calories

79 Calories • 3 gm Fat • 4 gm Protein • 9 gm Carbohydrate • 288 mg Sodium • 125 mg Calcium • 1 gm Fiber

DIABETIC: 2 Vegetable • ½ Meat

Carrots Supreme

It's just amazing how much kitchen magic you can work using tiny amounts of flavoring in a vegetable dish like this low-calorie carrot concoction! It's savory and sweet all at once, and delivers great taste as well as good nutrition. ☻ Serves 4 (scant 1 cup)

4 cups sliced carrots

2 cups hot water

½ cup diced onion

2 tablespoons Hormel Bacon Bits

¼ teaspoon black pepper

2 tablespoons Cary's Sugar Free Maple Syrup

In a medium saucepan, cook carrots in water for 10 minutes or until tender. Meanwhile, in a large saucepan sprayed with butter-flavored cooking spray, sauté onion for 5 minutes or until tender. Stir in bacon bits and black pepper. Drain carrots and return to saucepan. Mash well with potato masher or electric mixer. Stir in maple syrup. Add carrots to onion mixture. Mix well to combine. Continue cooking until heated through. Serve at once.

Each serving equals:

HE: 2¼ Vegetable • 18 Optional Calories

65 Calories • 1 gm Fat • 3 gm Protein • 11 gm Carbohydrate • 204 mg Sodium • 41 mg Calcium • 3 gm Fiber

DIABETIC: 2 Vegetable

Creamed Peas and Carrots

Creamed vegetable dishes always seem so old-timey and cozy to me, and this one will dazzle you with its smooth richness! If your family is bored with those same old peas and carrots they've always eaten, tickle their taste buds with this easy-cook recipe.

● Serves 6 (full ½ cup)

> 1½ cups frozen sliced carrots
> 1½ cups hot water
> 1½ cups frozen peas
> 1½ cups (one 12-fluid-ounce can) Carnation Evaporated Skim Milk
> 3 tablespoons all-purpose flour
> 1 teaspoon dried parsley flakes
> ¼ teaspoon lemon pepper
> ½ teaspoon Sugar Twin or Sprinkle Sweet

In a medium saucepan, cook carrots in water for 15 minutes. Add peas. Mix well to combine. Continue cooking for 5 minutes. Drain. In a covered jar, combine evaporated skim milk and flour. Shake well to blend. Pour mixture into same saucepan now sprayed with butter-flavored cooking spray. Stir in parsley flakes, lemon pepper, and sugar substitute. Cook for 2 to 3 minutes, stirring constantly. Add peas and carrots to milk mixture. Mix well to combine. Lower heat and simmer for 10 minutes or until mixture thickens, stirring often.

Each serving equals:

HE: ⅔ Bread • ½ Vegetable • ½ Skim Milk

100 Calories • 0 gm Fat • 7 gm Protein •
18 gm Carbohydrate • 91 mg Sodium •
205 mg Calcium • 2 gm Fiber

DIABETIC: ½ Starch • ½ Vegetable •
½ Skim Milk *or* 1 Starch/Carbohydrate • ½ Vegetable

Stewed Tomatoes with Bread Cubes

The chunks of bread mixed into this tangy-sweet tomato dish make it extra-hearty, but it's definitely a recipe to warm the hearts of everyone who tries it! If you find this dish a little too sweet, see if halving the sweetener will perfectly please your palate.

◑ Serves 4 (¾ cup)

> 3½ cups (two 14½-ounce cans) stewed tomatoes, undrained
> 1 teaspoon dried parsley flakes
> ½ teaspoon black pepper
> 2 teaspoons Sugar Twin or Sprinkle Sweet
> 2 slices stale reduced-calorie white bread, cut into cubes

In a large saucepan, combine undrained stewed tomatoes, parsley flakes, and black pepper. Bring mixture to a boil. Stir in sugar substitute. Add bread cubes. Mix gently to combine. Lower heat and simmer for 10 minutes, or until mixture is heated through, stirring often.

Each serving equals:

HE: 1¾ Vegetable • ¼ Bread • 1 Optional Calorie

80 Calories • 0 gm Fat • 3 gm Protein •
17 gm Carbohydrate • 688 mg Sodium •
122 mg Calcium • 3 gm Fiber

DIABETIC: 2 Vegetable

Cauliflower au Gratin in Tomato Sauce

Cauliflower just seems to go hand-in-hand with luscious hot cheese sauce, don't you agree? And you'll be pleased to discover how a blend of spices will give this easy-to-fix dish the taste of something fancy! ❍ Serves 6 (½ cup)

4 cups frozen cut cauliflower
2 cups water
1 (10¾-ounce) can Healthy Request Tomato Soup
½ teaspoon dried minced garlic
2 teaspoons dried parsley flakes
1 teaspoon prepared mustard
¼ teaspoon lemon pepper
⅔ cup (2¼ ounces) shredded Kraft reduced-fat Cheddar cheese

In a medium saucepan, cook cauliflower in water until tender. Drain. In a large skillet, combine tomato soup, garlic, parsley flakes, mustard, and lemon pepper. Mix well to combine. Stir in Cheddar cheese and cauliflower. Continue cooking until cheese melts, stirring often.

Each serving equals:

HE: 1⅓ Vegetable • ½ Protein • ¼ Slider • 10 Optional Calories

78 Calories • 2 gm Fat • 5 gm Protein • 10 gm Carbohydrate • 271 mg Sodium • 91 mg Calcium • 2 gm Fiber

DIABETIC: 1½ Vegetable • ½ Starch

Tomato Garden Dish

Here's a spectacular summertime treat that takes something utterly delectable and makes it even better! Use your freshest, ripest tomatoes from the garden or farmstand, then just stand back and enjoy the aroma filling your house as this dish bakes. You won't have to ring the dinner bell the night you put this on the menu!

◐ Serves 4

3 cups peeled fresh tomato wedges
¾ cup (3 ounces) shredded Kraft reduced-fat Cheddar cheese
¾ cup (3 ounces) dried fine bread crumbs
1 cup chopped green bell pepper
½ cup chopped onion
¼ cup Kraft Fat-Free Italian Dressing

Preheat oven to 300 degrees. Spray an 8-by-8-inch baking dish with olive oil–flavored cooking spray. In a large bowl, combine tomatoes, Cheddar cheese, bread crumbs, green pepper, and onion. Add Italian dressing. Mix gently to combine. Pour mixture into prepared baking dish. Bake for 45 to 50 minutes or until vegetables are tender. Divide into 4 servings.

Each serving equals:

HE: 2¼ Vegetable • 1 Protein • 1 Bread •
8 Optional Calories

185 Calories • 5 gm Fat • 10 gm Protein •
25 gm Carbohydrate • 525 mg Sodium •
209 mg Calcium • 3 gm Fiber

DIABETIC: 2 Vegetable • 1 Meat • 1 Starch

Mushroom-Scalloped Potatoes

Making heart-healthy scalloped potatoes seemed impossible for a long time—in fact, until those wonderful people figured out how to make fat-free sour cream and healthy creamy soups! This is a lovely dish to serve company because it looks so pretty and tastes so rich.

☻ Serves 6

> 4 cups (20 ounces) thinly sliced raw potatoes
> 1 cup thinly sliced onion
> 1 (10¾-ounce) can Healthy Request Cream of Mushroom Soup
> ½ cup Land O Lakes no-fat sour cream
> ¼ teaspoon black pepper
> 1 teaspoon dried parsley flakes

Preheat oven to 375 degrees. Spray an 8-by-8-inch baking dish with butter-flavored cooking spray. Layer half of potatoes in prepared dish and cover with half of onion. In a small bowl, combine mushroom soup, sour cream, black pepper, and parsley flakes. Spoon half of mixture over top. Repeat layers. Bake for 1¼ to 1½ hours or until potatoes are tender. Place baking dish on a wire rack and let set for 5 minutes. Divide into 6 servings.

Each serving equals:

HE: ⅔ Bread • ⅓ Vegetable • ½ Slider •
8 Optional Calories

---

113 Calories • 1 gm Fat • 3 gm Protein •
23 gm Carbohydrate • 232 mg Sodium •
68 mg Calcium • 2 gm Fiber

DIABETIC: 1½ Starch

Potato-Tomato au Gratin ❄

Don't dishes topped with baked cheese just make your taste buds stand up and cheer? This one is especially savory and full of flavor, but you don't have to save this luscious concoction for special occasions. It's perfect for a cozy family supper on a winter night.

⊙ Serves 6

4 cups (20 ounces) diced raw potatoes
¾ cup finely chopped onion
1½ cups (6 ounces) shredded Kraft reduced-fat Cheddar cheese
1 (10¾-ounce) can Healthy Request Tomato Soup
⅓ cup water
1 teaspoon dried parsley flakes

Preheat oven to 350 degrees. Spray an 8-by-8-inch baking dish with butter-flavored cooking spray. Place potatoes, onion, and Cheddar cheese in prepared baking dish. Mix well to combine. In a small bowl, combine tomato soup, water, and parsley flakes. Stir soup mixture into potato mixture. Cover with foil and bake for 45 to 50 minutes. Remove foil and continue baking for 25 to 30 minutes. Place baking dish on a wire rack and let set for 5 minutes. Divide into 6 servings.

Each serving equals:

HE: 1⅓ Protein • ⅔ Bread • ¼ Vegetable •
¼ Slider • 10 Optional Calories

178 Calories • 6 gm Fat • 10 gm Protein •
21 gm Carbohydrate • 419 mg Sodium •
221 mg Calcium • 2 gm Fiber

DIABETIC: 1½ Starch • 1 Meat

Veggie Trio Crock-Pot

Ever notice how good the vegetables taste in a bowl of beef stew? Well, you'll be amazed to find that old-fashioned flavor in this simple slow cooker recipe—but without the beef! Here, a little beef broth and lots of oh-so-slow baking time brews up a richly satisfying veggie dish that the whole family will love.

◔ Serves 4 (1 full cup)

> 3 cups (15 ounces) sliced raw potatoes
> 3 cups sliced carrots
> ½ cup chopped onion
> 1¾ cups (one 14½-ounce can) Swanson Beef Broth

In a slow cooker container, combine potatoes, carrots, and onion. Pour beef broth evenly over top. Cover and cook on HIGH for 4 to 6 hours. Mix well before serving.

Each serving equals:

HE: 1¾ Vegetable • ¾ Bread • 9 Optional Calories

109 Calories • 1 gm Fat • 3 gm Protein •
22 gm Carbohydrate • 410 mg Sodium •
38 mg Calcium • 3 gm Fiber

DIABETIC: 1½ Vegetable • 1 Starch

Beans and More Beans ❄

Everywhere I go, I get requests for healthy Crock-Pot cuisine from busy working people who love using their pots to make healthy food that doesn't need to be watched during cooking. Here's a truly comforting and very high fiber dish that tastes of so much old-fashioned flavor, you'll think that Grandma made it!

○ Serves 8 (¾ cup)

10 ounces (one 16-ounce can) pinto beans, rinsed and drained
10 ounces (one 16-ounce can) great northern beans, rinsed and drained
10 ounces (one 16-ounce can) butter beans, rinsed and drained
10 ounces (one 16-ounce can) red kidney beans, rinsed and drained
2 tablespoons Brown Sugar Twin
¾ cup chopped onion
½ cup chopped green bell pepper
¼ cup Heinz Light Harvest Ketchup or any reduced-sodium ketchup
1¾ cups (one 14½-ounce can) stewed tomatoes, undrained

In a slow cooker container, combine pinto beans, great northern beans, butter beans, and kidney beans. Add Brown Sugar Twin, onion, green pepper, ketchup, and undrained stewed tomatoes. Mix well to combine. Cover and cook on LOW for 6 to 8 hours. Mix well before serving.

Each serving equals:

HE: 2½ Protein • ¾ Vegetable • 9 Optional Calories

172 Calories • 0 gm Fat • 10 gm Protein •
33 gm Carbohydrate • 288 mg Sodium •
94 mg Calcium • 9 gm Fiber

DIABETIC: 2 Starch • 1½ Meat • ½ Vegetable

He-Man Baked Beans

There's no more popular man-pleaser than baked beans, but the traditional preparation is both high in fat and calories. I didn't let that discourage me, however, but tested up a storm until I could serve the man in my house a dish he'd truly love!

○ Serves 6

> 20 ounces (two 16-ounce cans) great northern beans, rinsed and drained
> ½ cup chopped onion
> ½ cup chunky salsa (mild, medium, or hot)
> 1 (10¾-ounce) can Healthy Request Tomato Soup
> 2 tablespoons Brown Sugar Twin
> ¼ teaspoon black pepper
> 2 tablespoons Hormel Bacon Bits

Preheat oven to 350 degrees. Spray an 8-by-8-inch baking dish with butter-flavored cooking spray. In a large bowl, combine great northern beans, onion, salsa, and tomato soup. Stir in Brown Sugar Twin, black pepper, and bacon bits. Mix well to combine. Pour mixture into prepared baking dish. Bake for 60 minutes. Place baking dish on a wire rack and let set for 3 to 4 minutes. Divide into 6 servings.

Each serving equals:

HE: 1⅔ Protein • ⅓ Vegetable • ½ Slider

161 Calories • 1 gm Fat • 10 gm Protein • 28 gm Carbohydrate • 312 mg Sodium • 99 mg Calcium • 6 gm Fiber

DIABETIC: 2 Starch • 1 Meat

Crock-Pot Party Beans

Crock-Pots were born to make scrumptious bean dishes, and I enjoy coming up with sparkling new ways to prepare this old but popular standby. Just think of it—for hours and hours, your beans will be mingling with tangy ham and spicy salsa. Mmm-hmm!

☻ Serves 6 (1 full cup)

> *30 ounces (three 16-ounce cans) great northern beans, rinsed and drained*
>
> *½ cup chopped onion*
>
> *1 scant cup (4.5 ounces) finely diced Dubuque 97% fat-free ham or any extra-lean ham*
>
> *½ cup chunky salsa (mild, medium, or hot)*
>
> *1¾ cups (one 15-ounce can) Hunt's Tomato Sauce*
>
> *2 tablespoons Sugar Twin or Sprinkle Sweet*
>
> *2 tablespoons Brown Sugar Twin*
>
> *¼ teaspoon black pepper*

In a slow cooker container, combine great northern beans, onion, and ham. Add salsa, tomato sauce, sugar substitute, Brown Sugar Twin, and black pepper. Mix well to combine. Cover and cook on LOW for 8 hours. Mix well before serving.

Each serving equals:

HE: 3 Protein • 1⅓ Vegetable • 3 Optional Calories

213 Calories • 1 gm Fat • 16 gm Protein •
35 gm Carbohydrate • 723 mg Sodium •
126 mg Calcium • 9 gm Fiber

DIABETIC: 2 Starch • 1½ Meat • 1½ Vegetable

Main Dishes

Macaroni Cheese Bake

Is macaroni and cheese as popular at your house as it is at mine? I'm not surprised! This version lets you bake this cheesy favorite until the top is wonderfully crusty and brown, just the way most men and kids like it best. ● Serves 2

⅔ cup Carnation Nonfat Dry Milk Powder
½ cup water
2 teaspoons reduced-calorie margarine
¾ cup (3 ounces) shredded Kraft reduced-fat Cheddar cheese
1 cup hot cooked elbow macaroni, rinsed and drained

Preheat oven to 350 degrees. In a medium saucepan, combine dry milk powder, water, and margarine. Cook over medium heat until margarine melts, stirring often. Add Cheddar cheese and macaroni. Mix well to combine. Evenly spoon mixture into two (12-ounce) ovenproof custard dishes. Place custard dishes on a baking sheet. Bake for 30 minutes. Place baking sheet on a wire rack and let set for 2 to 3 minutes.

HINT: ⅔ cup uncooked macaroni usually cooks to about 1 cup.

Each serving equals:

HE: 2 Protein • 1 Skim Milk • 1 Bread • ½ Fat

305 Calories • 9 gm Fat • 23 gm Protein • 33 gm Carbohydrate • 532 mg Sodium • 587 mg Calcium • 0 gm Fiber

DIABETIC: 2 Meat • 1 Skim Milk • 1 Starch • ½ Fat

Stroganoff Macaroni and Cheese

I closed my eyes and imagined what might happen if traditional American mac and cheese decided to mingle with a little sour cream and a few mushrooms. The result? A truly fabulous blend of cuisines and flavors, baked up so delectably fragrant that everyone will be smacking their lips until dinner is served! It's elegant *and* easy. ☻ Serves 4

> 1 (10¾-ounce) can Healthy Request Cream of Mushroom Soup
> 1½ cups (6 ounces) shredded Kraft reduced-fat Cheddar cheese
> ½ cup (one 2.5-ounce jar) sliced mushrooms, drained
> ⅓ cup Land O Lakes no-fat sour cream
> 1 teaspoon dried parsley flakes
> ¼ teaspoon black pepper
> 2 cups hot cooked elbow macaroni, rinsed and drained

Preheat oven to 350 degrees. Spray an 8-by-8-inch baking dish with butter-flavored cooking spray. In a medium saucepan, combine mushroom soup and Cheddar cheese. Cook over medium heat until cheese melts, stirring constantly. Remove from heat. Stir in mushrooms, sour cream, parsley flakes, and black pepper. Add macaroni. Mix well to combine. Pour mixture into prepared baking dish. Bake for 30 minutes. Place baking dish on a wire rack and let set for 5 minutes. Divide into 4 servings.

HINT: 1⅓ cups uncooked macaroni usually cooks to about 2 cups.

Each serving equals:

> HE: 2 Protein • 1 Bread • ¼ Vegetable • ¾ Slider • 1 Optional Calorie
>
> ───────────────────────────
>
> 277 Calories • 9 gm Fat • 17 gm Protein • 32 gm Carbohydrate • 800 mg Sodium • 386 mg Calcium • 1 gm Fiber
>
> ───────────────────────────
>
> DIABETIC: 2 Meat • 2 Starch

Italian Macaroni and Beans ❄

Are you trying to eat more meatless main dishes at your house? Then you may have heard the expression "a complete protein." This means combining two healthy foods—in this case, beans and pasta—to provide all the nutrition you might ordinarily get from meat dishes. But anyone who dines on this tasty baked entree will be more interested in just how delicious it is! ☻ Serves 4

½ cup chopped onion

1½ cups chopped unpeeled zucchini

10 ounces (one 16-ounce can) navy beans, rinsed and drained

1¾ cups (one 15-ounce can) Hunt's Tomato Sauce

1 teaspoon Italian seasoning

½ teaspoon dried minced garlic

2 cups hot cooked elbow macaroni, rinsed and drained

¼ cup (¾ ounce) grated Kraft fat-free Parmesan cheese ☆

Preheat oven to 350 degrees. Spray an 8-by-8-inch baking dish with butter-flavored cooking spray. In a large skillet sprayed with olive oil–flavored cooking spray, sauté onion and zucchini for 5 minutes or until tender. Stir in navy beans, tomato sauce, Italian seasoning, garlic, macaroni, and 2 tablespoons Parmesan cheese. Pour mixture into prepared baking dish. Evenly sprinkle remaining Parmesan cheese over top. Bake for 30 minutes. Place baking dish on a wire rack and let set for 5 minutes. Divide into 4 servings.

HINT: 1⅓ cups uncooked macaroni usually cooks to about 2 cups.

Each serving equals:

HE: 2¾ Vegetable • 1½ Protein • 1 Bread

241 Calories • 1 gm Fat • 12 gm Protein •
46 gm Carbohydrate • 816 mg Sodium •
66 mg Calcium • 11 gm Fiber

DIABETIC: 3 Vegetable • 2 Starch • 1 Meat

Confetti Spaghetti

There's something so satisfying about food that looks as colorful and hearty as it tastes, and this recipe is no exception. The cheesy sauce is downright yummy, and the pile of tasty veggies "on top of spaghetti," as the song goes, will make your kids just smack their lips when dinner is served! ☺ Serves 4

> 2½ cups frozen carrot, broccoli, and cauliflower blend
> 1 cup hot water
> ½ cup finely chopped onion
> ½ cup chopped fresh mushrooms
> 1½ cups (one 12-fluid-ounce can) Carnation Evaporated Skim Milk
> 3 tablespoons all-purpose flour
> 1 teaspoon Italian seasoning
> ¾ cup (3 ounces) shredded Kraft reduced-fat Cheddar cheese
> 2 cups hot cooked spaghetti, rinsed and drained
> ¼ cup (¾ ounce) grated Kraft fat-free Parmesan cheese

In a medium saucepan, cook frozen vegetables in water for 5 minutes or until tender. Drain. Meanwhile, in a large skillet sprayed with butter-flavored cooking spray, sauté onion and mushrooms for 5 minutes or until tender. Stir in drained vegetables. In a covered jar, combine evaporated skim milk and flour. Shake well to blend. Pour flour mixture into skillet with vegetables. Add Italian seasoning and Cheddar cheese. Mix well to combine. Lower heat and simmer for 10 minutes or until mixture thickens and cheese melts, stirring often. For each serving, place ½ cup cooked spaghetti on a plate, spoon about 1 cup vegetable mixture over spaghetti, and sprinkle 1 tablespoon Parmesan cheese over top.

HINTS: 1. 1½ cups broken uncooked spaghetti usually cooks to about 2 cups.
2. 1 cup carrots, ¾ cup broccoli, and ¾ cup cauliflower may be used in place of blended vegetables.

Each serving equals:

HE: 1¾ Vegetable • 1¼ Bread • 1¼ Protein •
¾ Skim Milk

---

317 Calories • 5 gm Fat • 20 gm Protein •
48 gm Carbohydrate • 448 mg Sodium •
471 mg Calcium • 4 gm Fiber

DIABETIC: 2 Vegetable • 1½ Starch • 1 Meat •

1 Skim Milk

Dijon Green Beans and Pasta ❄

I like to think of Dijon mustard as one of my favorite "secret ingredients," and this recipe will show you just why. Only a teaspoon gives this appetizing entree an astonishing amount of flavor. I won't promise that your family will start dancing the can-can when you serve it, but you know, they just might!

❍   Serves 4 (1 cup)

>   ½ cup finely chopped onion
>   1 (10¾-ounce) can Healthy Request Cream of Mushroom Soup
>   1 teaspoon Dijon mustard
>   1 teaspoon dried parsley flakes
>   ¼ teaspoon black pepper
>   2 cups (one 16-ounce can) French-style green beans, rinsed and
>   drained
>   2 cups hot cooked rotini pasta, rinsed and drained
>   ¾ cup (3 ounces) shredded Kraft reduced-fat Cheddar cheese

In a large skillet sprayed with butter-flavored cooking spray, sauté onion for 5 minutes or until tender. Add mushroom soup, mustard, parsley flakes, and black pepper. Mix well to combine. Stir in green beans, rotini pasta, and Cheddar cheese. Lower heat and simmer for 15 minutes or until cheese melts, stirring often.

HINT: 1½ cups uncooked rotini pasta usually cooks to about
        2 cups.

Each serving equals:

> HE: 1¼ Vegetable • 1 Bread • 1 Protein • ½ Slider •
> 1 Optional Calorie
>
> ---
>
> 226 Calories • 6 gm Fat • 11 gm Protein •
> 32 gm Carbohydrate • 528 mg Sodium •
> 232 mg Calcium • 2 gm Fiber
>
> ---
>
> DIABETIC: 1½ Starch • 1 Vegetable • 1 Meat

Mashed Potato Spinach Bake

Here's an inventive vegetarian main dish that is so soothing and satisfying, no one will notice that you've left out the meat! I think you'll be pleased to discover that the dry milk powder and yogurt give the mashed potato topping an irresistible creaminess that's as rich in calcium as it is in flavor. ○ Serves 6

2½ cups water
2 cups (4½ ounces) instant potato flakes
⅓ cup Carnation Nonfat Dry Milk Powder
¾ cup Yoplait plain fat-free yogurt
1 teaspoon Italian seasoning
½ cup (one 2.5-ounce jar) sliced mushrooms, drained
1 (10-ounce) package frozen chopped spinach, thawed and thoroughly drained
1½ cups (6 ounces) shredded Kraft reduced-fat Cheddar cheese

Preheat oven to 375 degrees. Spray an 8-by-8-inch baking dish with butter-flavored cooking spray. In a large saucepan, bring water to a boil. Remove from heat. Add potato flakes and dry milk powder. Mix well using a fork. Stir in yogurt and Italian seasoning. Add mushrooms, spinach, and Cheddar cheese. Mix well to combine. Spread mixture into prepared baking dish. Bake for 30 to 35 minutes. Place baking dish on a wire rack and let set for 5 minutes. Divide into 6 servings.

Each serving equals:

HE: 1⅓ Protein • 1 Bread • ⅔ Vegetable • ⅓ Skim Milk

---

173 Calories • 5 gm Fat • 13 gm Protein • 19 gm Carbohydrate • 386 mg Sodium • 347 mg Calcium • 3 gm Fiber

---

DIABETIC: 1 Meat • 1 Starch • 1 Vegetable

Spinach Italian Pizza

Does homemade pizza seem like just too much trouble, especially when you can have it delivered pretty quickly? Ah, but you'd have to look far and wide for this special pizza with a topping that's richer than rich! With a blend of three cheeses and tangy dressing, combined with iron-rich spinach, you've got a great-tasting dish that's also really good for you! ☺ Serves 8

> 1 (11-ounce) can refrigerated Pillsbury French Loaf
> 1 (8-ounce) package Philadelphia fat-free cream cheese
> 2 tablespoons Kraft Fat-Free Italian Dressing
> 1/4 cup (3/4 ounce) grated Kraft fat-free Parmesan cheese
> 1/2 cup (one 2.5-ounce jar) sliced mushrooms, drained
> 1 (10-ounce) package frozen chopped spinach, thawed and well
>   drained
> 1 1/3 cups (4 1/2 ounces) shredded Kraft reduced-fat mozzarella cheese

Preheat oven to 400 degrees. Spray a rimmed 12-by-15-inch baking pan with olive oil–flavored cooking spray. Unroll French loaf and pat into prepared pan and up sides to form a rim. Bake for 5 minutes. Meanwhile, in a large bowl, stir cream cheese with a spoon until soft. Stir in Italian dressing, Parmesan cheese, and mushrooms. Add well-drained spinach. Mix well to combine. Evenly spread mixture over partially baked crust. Sprinkle mozzarella cheese evenly over top. Bake for 15 to 20 minutes or until crust is browned. Place pan on a wire rack and let set for 5 minutes. Divide into 8 servings.

Each serving equals:

> HE: 1 1/3 Protein • 1 Bread • 1/2 Vegetable •
> 5 Optional Calories
> _____
> 184 Calories • 4 gm Fat • 14 gm Protein •
> 23 gm Carbohydrate • 683 mg Sodium •
> 144 mg Calcium • 2 gm Fiber
> _____
> DIABETIC: 1 1/2 Meat • 1 Starch • 1 Vegetable

Chili Corn-Stuffed Peppers

Stuffed peppers are an American classic, especially here in the Midwest, but you don't want to get stuck in a rut, do you? I didn't think so. Why not try this tempting blend of flavors on your family tonight, and see if they notice how newly tasty this old-timey dish has become? ☻ Serves 4

10 ounces (one 16-ounce can) pinto beans, rinsed and drained
½ cup frozen whole-kernel corn, thawed
1 cup (one 8-ounce can) Hunt's Tomato Sauce
1 teaspoon chili seasoning
4 (medium-sized) green bell peppers
2 cups hot water
⅓ cup (1½ ounces) shredded Kraft reduced-fat Cheddar cheese

Preheat oven to 350 degrees. In a large skillet sprayed with olive oil–flavored cooking spray, combine pinto beans, corn, tomato sauce, and chili seasoning. Cook over low heat while preparing green peppers, stirring occasionally. Cut top off green peppers and remove membrane. Place peppers in a large saucepan with water. Cook over medium heat for 10 minutes. Drain. Place green peppers in an 8-by-8-inch baking dish. Stir Cheddar cheese into bean mixture. Spoon about ½ cup bean mixture into each green pepper. Bake for 30 minutes.

HINT: Thaw corn by placing in a colander and rinsing under hot water for one minute.

Each serving equals:

HE: 2 Vegetable • 1¾ Protein • ¼ Bread

---

178 Calories • 2 gm Fat • 10 gm Protein •
30 gm Carbohydrate • 490 mg Sodium •
108 mg Calcium • 9 gm Fiber

DIABETIC: 2 Vegetable • 1 Meat • 1 Starch

Calzone Roll-Ups

These baked Italian savory pastries are a take-out favorite across the nation, but now you can bring that wonderful flavor home with this dish that's as fun to prepare as it is to eat! With three cheeses to delight the pickiest eaters, these roll-ups are great for a teen party.

◐ Serves 6

> 1 (11-ounce) can refrigerated Pillsbury French Loaf
> 1¾ cups (one 15-ounce can) Hunt's Tomato Sauce ☆
> 1½ teaspoons Italian seasoning ☆
> 2 teaspoons Sugar Twin or Sprinkle Sweet ☆
> ¼ cup (¾ ounce) grated Kraft fat-free Parmesan cheese
> ¾ cup (3 ounces) shredded Kraft reduced-fat Cheddar cheese ☆
> ¾ cup (3 ounces) shredded Kraft reduced-fat mozzarella cheese ☆
> ⅓ cup (1½ ounces) sliced ripe olives
> ½ cup (one 2.5-ounce jar) sliced mushrooms, drained

Preheat oven to 350 degrees. Spray a baking sheet with butter-flavored cooking spray. Remove French loaf from container but leave rolled up. Using a very sharp knife, evenly cut rolled loaf into 6 pieces. In a small bowl, combine ½ cup tomato sauce, 1 teaspoon Italian seasoning, 1 teaspoon sugar substitute, and Parmesan cheese. Gently unroll each piece of dough. Spread a full tablespoon of mixture on each strip of dough. In a small bowl, combine ¼ cup Cheddar cheese and ¼ cup mozzarella cheese. Evenly sprinkle cheese mixture over tomato sauce mixture. Gently reroll strips. Place roll-ups on prepared baking sheet. Lightly spray tops with butter-flavored cooking spray. Bake for 22 to 25 minutes. Ten minutes before roll-ups are through baking, combine remaining 1¼ cups tomato sauce, remaining ½ teaspoon Italian seasoning, and remaining 1 teaspoon sugar substitute in a medium saucepan. Stir in olives and mushrooms. Simmer over medium-low heat. Meanwhile, in a small bowl, combine remaining Cheddar and mozzarella cheeses. For each serving, place one roll-up on a plate, spoon ⅓ cup sauce over roll-up, and sprinkle about 2 tablespoons cheese mixture over top. Serve at once.

Each serving equals:

HE: 1½ Protein • 1⅓ Bread • 1⅓ Vegetable •
¼ Fat • 1 Optional Calorie

247 Calories • 7 gm Fat • 15 gm Protein •
31 gm Carbohydrate • 1,224 mg Sodium •
213 mg Calcium • 3 gm Fiber

DIABETIC: 1½ Meat • 1½ Starch • 1 Vegetable

Cheesy Tuna Garden Skillet

Tired of the same old ways to fix tuna, but interested in trying something fresh and new? Here's a cozy-warm dish that cooks up quickly, is rich in cheesy-creamy flavor, and truly warms the cockles of your family's hearts. Enjoy! ☻ Serves 6 (1 cup)

> 1 (6-ounce) can white tuna, packed in water, drained and flaked
> 1 (10¾-ounce) can Healthy Request Cream of Mushroom Soup
> ⅓ cup skim milk
> ¾ cup (3 ounces) shredded Kraft reduced-fat Cheddar cheese
> ¼ cup (¾ ounce) grated Kraft fat-free Parmesan cheese
> 1 teaspoon dried parsley flakes
> ¼ teaspoon black pepper
> 2 cups (one 16-ounce can) sliced carrots, rinsed and drained
> 2 cups (one 16-ounce can) French-style green beans, rinsed and drained
> 2 cups hot cooked noodles, rinsed and drained

In a large skillet, combine tuna, mushroom soup, and skim milk. Stir in Cheddar cheese, Parmesan cheese, parsley flakes, and black pepper. Cook over medium heat until cheeses melt, stirring often. Add carrots and green beans. Mix well to combine. Stir in noodles. Lower heat and simmer for 15 minutes or until mixture is heated through, stirring often.

HINT: 1¾ cups uncooked noodles usually cooks to about 2 cups.

Each serving equals:

HE: 1⅓ Protein • 1⅓ Vegetable • ⅔ Bread • ¼ Slider • 13 Optional Calories

209 Calories • 5 gm Fat • 17 gm Protein • 24 gm Carbohydrate • 505 mg Sodium • 185 mg Calcium • 3 gm Fiber

DIABETIC: 2 Meat • 1½ Vegetable • 1 Starch

Tuna à la Rice

Canned tuna is a great source of healthy protein, but it's easy to get into the habit of using it only for sandwiches or tuna noodle casserole. Here's a creamy rice dish that beautifully features this flavorful fish. You'll be astonished how thick the sauce gets!

Serves 4 (1 cup)

2 cups skim milk

3 tablespoons all-purpose flour

½ cup (4 ounces) Philadelphia fat-free cream cheese

1 cup frozen peas, thawed

1 (6-ounce) can white tuna, packed in water, drained and flaked

1 teaspoon dried parsley flakes

¼ cup (one 2-ounce jar) chopped pimiento, drained

¼ teaspoon black pepper

1 cup (3 ounces) uncooked Minute Rice

In a covered jar, combine skim milk and flour. Shake well to blend. Pour mixture into a large skillet sprayed with butter-flavored cooking spray. Stir in cream cheese. Cook over medium heat until mixture starts to thicken, stirring constantly. Add peas, tuna, parsley flakes, pimiento, and black pepper. Mix well to combine. Continue cooking just until mixture starts to boil. Remove from heat. Stir in uncooked rice. Cover and let set for 5 minutes. Fluff with fork before serving.

HINT: Thaw peas by placing in a colander and rinsing under hot water for one minute.

Each serving equals:

HE: 1½ Bread • 1¼ Protein • ½ Skim Milk

---

205 Calories • 1 gm Fat • 23 gm Protein •
26 gm Carbohydrate • 381 mg Sodium •
171 mg Calcium • 2 gm Fiber

DIABETIC: 2 Starch • 1½ Meat *or* 1½ Starch •
1½ Meat • ½ Skim Milk

Italian Shrimp Pasta

Fast and fabulous—that's what you'll say once you taste this sensational seafood pasta dish that's ready in just minutes! It's a thrifty dish, too, since only one small can of shrimp or fish serves four—and satisfies them too. ☻ Serves 4 (1 cup)

1 (10¾-ounce) can Healthy Request Tomato Soup
1 teaspoon Italian seasoning
¼ cup (¾ ounce) grated Kraft fat-free Parmesan cheese
1 (4.5-ounce drained weight) can tiny shrimp, rinsed and drained
2 cups hot cooked rotini pasta, rinsed and drained

In a large skillet, combine tomato soup and Italian seasoning. Cook over medium heat for 5 minutes or until heated through, stirring often. Stir in Parmesan cheese. Add shrimp and rotini pasta. Mix well to combine. Lower heat and continue simmering for 5 minutes or until mixture is heated through, stirring occasionally.

HINTS: 1. 1½ cups uncooked rotini pasta usually cooks to about 2 cups.
2. 1 (6-ounce) can tuna, packed in water, drained and flaked, may be used in place of the canned shrimp.

Each serving equals:

HE: 1⅓ Protein • 1 Bread • ½ Slider •
5 Optional Calories

202 Calories • 2 gm Fat • 12 gm Protein •
34 gm Carbohydrate • 391 mg Sodium •
30 mg Calcium • 2 gm Fiber

DIABETIC: 2 Starch • 1 Meat

Stovetop Chicken and Broccoli ❄

This dish is extra-easy for those evenings when time is at a real premium. The macaroni cooks along with the rest of the ingredients, and the sauce couldn't be creamier! When everyone's in a hurry but you've still got to eat well, choose this recipe—and you've chosen good health! (Come on, Cliff, give it a try. . . .)

☻ Serves 4 (1 cup)

> 1⅓ cups (3 ounces) uncooked elbow macaroni
> 2 cups frozen cut broccoli, partially thawed
> 2 cups water
> 1 (10¾-ounce) can Healthy Request Cream of Broccoli Soup
> ½ cup skim milk
> ¼ teaspoon black pepper
> 1 cup (5 ounces) diced cooked chicken breast

In a large saucepan, combine uncooked macaroni, broccoli, and water. Cook over medium heat about 10 minutes or until both macaroni and broccoli are tender. Drain. Return to saucepan. Add broccoli soup, skim milk, and black pepper. Mix well to combine. Stir in chicken. Lower heat and simmer for 5 minutes or until mixture is heated through, stirring occasionally.

HINT: If you don't have leftovers, purchase a chunk of cooked chicken breast from your local deli.

Each serving equals:

HE: 1¼ Protein • 1 Bread • 1 Vegetable • ½ Slider •
13 Optional Calories

---

199 Calories • 3 gm Fat • 17 gm Protein •
26 gm Carbohydrate • 371 mg Sodium •
151 mg Calcium • 2 gm Fiber

DIABETIC: 1½ Starch • 1 Meat • 1 Vegetable

Chicken-Apple Swiss Bake ✳

Think how good a slab of cheese tastes with warm apple pie. Now, think about how luscious baked chicken can be. Is your mouth watering yet? Oh, good—you're ready to stir up this truly inviting dish that combines so many good tastes into one amazing feast!

◗ Serves 6

3 full cups (4½ ounces) dried bread cubes
2 cups (4 small) cored, unpeeled, and diced cooking apples
¾ cup chopped celery
1 cup unsweetened apple juice ☆
4 (¾-ounce) slices Kraft reduced-fat Swiss cheese, shredded
8 ounces skinned and boned uncooked chicken breast, cut into
*   12 pieces*
1 (10¾-ounce) can Healthy Request Cream of Chicken Soup
1 teaspoon dried parsley flakes

Preheat oven to 350 degrees. Spray a 9-by-13-inch baking dish with butter-flavored cooking spray. In a large bowl, combine bread cubes, apples, and celery. Add ¾ cup apple juice. Mix gently to combine. (Mixture will be somewhat dry.) Pat mixture into prepared baking dish. Evenly sprinkle Swiss cheese over top. Place chicken pieces on top of cheese. In a small bowl, combine chicken soup, remaining ¼ cup apple juice, and parsley flakes. Spoon mixture evenly over top. Bake for 50 minutes. Divide into 6 servings.

HINT: Brownberry unseasoned toasted bread cubes work great.

Each serving equals:

HE: 1⅔ Protein • 1 Fruit • 1 Bread • ¼ Vegetable •
¼ Slider • 10 Optional Calories

231 Calories • 3 gm Fat • 17 gm Protein •
34 gm Carbohydrate • 529 mg Sodium •
153 mg Calcium • 2 gm Fiber

DIABETIC: 1½ Meat • 1 Fruit • 1 Starch

Mexi-Chicken Lasagna Bake ❄

Some of my best-loved recipes invite the cuisines of two different nations to shake hands and come out smiling! This dish is sure to elicit a few "Bravos" and some shouts of "Olé!" when everyone gobbles it down.   ☻   Serves 4

½ cup chopped onion
1 (10¾-ounce) can Healthy Request Cream of Chicken Soup
1 cup chunky salsa (mild, medium, or hot)
2 cups hot cooked mini lasagna noodles, rinsed and drained☆
1 full cup (6 ounces) diced cooked chicken breast☆
¾ cup (3 ounces) shredded Kraft reduced-fat Cheddar cheese
¼ cup Land O Lakes no-fat sour cream

Preheat oven to 350 degrees. Spray an 8-by-8-inch baking dish with olive oil–flavored cooking spray. In a large skillet sprayed with olive oil–flavored cooking spray, sauté onion for 5 minutes or until tender. Stir in chicken soup and salsa. Spoon about ½ cup soup mixture into prepared baking dish. Layer half of noodles and chicken over soup mixture. Spoon half of remaining soup mixture over chicken. Repeat layers. Evenly sprinkle Cheddar cheese over top. Bake for 20 minutes. Place baking dish on a wire rack and let set for 5 minutes. Divide into 4 servings. When serving, top each with 1 tablespoon sour cream.

HINTS: 1. 1¾ cups uncooked lasagna noodles usually cooks to about 2 cups.
2. If you can't find mini lasagna noodles, use regular medium-width noodles.
3. If you don't have leftovers, purchase a chunk of cooked chicken breast from your local deli.

Each serving equals:

HE: 2½ Protein • 1 Bread • ¾ Vegetable • ¾ Slider

351 Calories • 7 gm Fat • 26 gm Protein •
46 gm Carbohydrate • 751 mg Sodium •
254 mg Calcium • 2 gm Fiber

DIABETIC: 2½ Starch • 2 Meat • 1 Vegetable

Creamed Chicken with Cornbread Shortcakes

Are you looking for something special to serve at a family brunch or festive late-night supper? This old-fashioned chicken dish might just fill the bill! When was the last time you served homemade cornbread like this—just laden with creamy chicken and veggies? This is definitely a "Grandma" dish, made heart-healthy and easy for today's busy families. ☻ Serves 6

¾ cup all-purpose flour

¼ cup (1½ ounces) yellow cornmeal

1 tablespoon Sugar Twin or Sprinkle Sweet

1 teaspoon baking powder

2 teaspoons dried onion flakes

1 tablespoon dried parsley flakes ☆

½ cup skim milk

1 egg or equivalent in egg substitute

2 tablespoons vegetable oil

1¼ cups water

¼ cup finely chopped onion

¾ cup finely chopped celery

1½ cups (8 ounces) diced cooked chicken breast

2 (10¾-ounce) cans Healthy Request Cream of Chicken Soup

⅓ cup Carnation Nonfat Dry Milk Powder

¼ teaspoon black pepper

Preheat oven to 400 degrees. Spray 6 wells of a muffin pan with butter-flavored cooking spray or line with paper liners. In a medium bowl, combine flour, cornmeal, sugar substitute, baking powder, onion flakes, and 2 teaspoons parsley flakes. Add skim milk, egg, and vegetable oil. Mix well to combine. Fill muffin wells a scant half full. Bake for 12 to 15 minutes or until a toothpick inserted in center of muffin comes out clean. Meanwhile, in a medium saucepan, combine water, onion, and celery. Bring mixture to a boil. Stir in chicken. Lower heat and simmer for 6 to 8 minutes, stirring occasionally. Add chicken soup, dry milk powder, black pepper, and remaining 1 teaspoon parsley flakes. Mix well to combine. Lower heat and continue to simmer until shortcakes are done. For each serving, place 1 shortcake on a plate and spoon about ¾ cup chicken mixture over top.

HINTS: 1. If you don't have leftovers, purchase a chunk of cooked chicken breast from your local deli.

2. Fill unused muffin wells with water. It protects the muffin tin and ensures even baking.

Each serving equals:

HE: 1½ Protein • 1 Bread • 1 Fat • ⅓ Vegetable •
¼ Skim Milk • ¾ Slider • 1 Optional Calorie

248 Calories • 8 gm Fat • 18 gm Protein •
26 gm Carbohydrate • 365 mg Sodium •
140 mg Calcium • 1 gm Fiber

DIABETIC: 1½ Meat • 1½ Starch • 1 Fat

Harvest Chicken Skillet

Here's a succulent summer supper that looks very pretty—and provides tons of good nutrition for very few calories! I prefer to use peeled tomatoes in this dish, but you could also try this with the skins on if you're especially rushed. What a festive way to celebrate your garden's tomato harvest! ☻ Serves 4

> 16 ounces skinned and boned uncooked chicken breast, cut into
>   24 pieces
> 1 (10¾-ounce) can Healthy Request Cream of Mushroom Soup
> 1 cup frozen whole-kernel corn, thawed
> ¼ cup skim milk
> ½ teaspoon dried minced garlic
> 1½ cups peeled and chopped fresh tomatoes
> 2 teaspoons dried parsley flakes
> 1 cup hot cooked rice

In a large skillet sprayed with butter-flavored cooking spray, brown chicken pieces. Add mushroom soup, corn, skim milk, and garlic. Mix well to combine. Lower heat, cover, and simmer for 10 minutes, stirring occasionally. Stir in tomatoes, parsley flakes, and rice. Re-cover and continue simmering for 10 minutes or until mixture is heated through, stirring occasionally.

HINTS: 1. ⅔ cup uncooked rice usually cooks to about 1 cup.
       2. Thaw corn by placing in a colander and rinsing under
          hot water for one minute.

Each serving equals:

HE: 3 Protein • 1 Bread • ¾ Vegetable • ½ Slider •
7 Optional Calories

---

259 Calories • 3 gm Fat • 30 gm Protein •
28 gm Carbohydrate • 392 mg Sodium •
93 mg Calcium • 2 gm Fiber

DIABETIC: 3 Meat • 1½ Starch • 1 Vegetable

Chicken Breast with Corn-Walnut Salsa

One of the true secrets of satisfying heart-healthy dining is blending lots of textures and tastes together so you don't miss the fat I've whisked out. This simple skillet supper tastes like something a fancy restaurant might serve up, but this crunchy and colorful combo is really down-home cooking with a little uptown flair.

Serves 4

> *16 ounces skinned and boned uncooked chicken breast, cut into 4 pieces*
> *½ cup chopped green bell pepper*
> *¼ cup (1 ounce) chopped walnuts*
> *¼ cup (one 2-ounce jar) chopped pimiento, undrained*
> *2 cups frozen whole-kernel corn, thawed*
> *½ cup Kraft Fat-Free Catalina Dressing*
> *½ teaspoon chili seasoning*

In a large skillet sprayed with butter-flavored cooking spray, cook chicken pieces for 4 minutes on each side. Remove chicken from skillet and cover to keep warm. In same skillet, sauté green pepper and walnuts for 5 minutes, stirring often. Stir in undrained pimiento, corn, Catalina dressing, and chili seasoning. Push chicken pieces into corn mixture. Lower heat, cover, and simmer for 4 to 6 minutes. For each serving, place 1 piece of chicken on a plate and spoon about ½ cup corn mixture over top.

HINT: Thaw corn by placing in a colander and rinsing under hot water for one minute.

Each serving equals:

HE: 3¼ Protein • 1 Bread • ½ Fat • ¼ Vegetable • ½ Slider • 10 Optional Calories

---

282 Calories • 6 gm Fat • 30 gm Protein • 27 gm Carbohydrate • 420 mg Sodium • 23 mg Calcium • 3 gm Fiber

---

DIABETIC: 3 Meat • 1½ Starch • 1 Fat

Chicken with Cashews in Plum Sauce

Cliff and I love to visit Chinese restaurants when we're on the road, but so many dishes that sound wonderful on the menu are very high in sugar and fat. Here's one tasty main dish I reinvented the Healthy Exchanges way, and I bet you'll agree it's a winner. I get a lot of mileage out of just a few nuts, but you won't feel deprived—and your heart will say "Thanks!" ❷ Serves 4

> 12 ounces skinned and boned uncooked chicken breast, cut into
>   24 pieces
> ¼ cup (1 ounce) chopped cashews
> ¼ cup plum spreadable fruit
> 1 teaspoon ground ginger
> 2 tablespoons Sugar Twin or Sprinkle Sweet
> 2 cups hot cooked rice
> ½ cup finely chopped green onion

In a large skillet sprayed with butter-flavored cooking spray, sauté chicken pieces for 5 minutes or until tender, stirring often. Stir in cashews. In a small bowl, combine spreadable fruit, ginger, and sugar substitute. Add to chicken mixture. Mix well to combine. Lower heat and simmer for 5 minutes, stirring often. For each serving, place ½ cup rice on plate, spoon about ½ cup chicken mixture over top, and garnish with 2 tablespoons green onion.

HINTS: 1. 1⅓ cups uncooked rice usually cooks to about 2 cups.
2. Grape or apricot spreadable fruit can be substituted for plum.

Each serving equals:

HE: 2½ Protein • 1 Fruit • 1 Bread • ½ Fat •
3 Optional Calories

265 Calories • 5 gm Fat • 23 gm Protein •
32 gm Carbohydrate • 113 mg Sodium •
24 mg Calcium • 1 gm Fiber

DIABETIC: 2½ Meat • 1 Fruit • 1 Starch • ½ Fat

Mexicalli-Turkey Stroganoff

This post-Thanksgiving skillet supper can be as tangy and spicy as your family likes it—just check the label on the salsa jar and then go to town! And if you haven't got leftovers, do what the Lunds do and pick up a chunk of roast turkey at your nearest deli or super-market. ● Serves 6

> 1½ cups (8 ounces) diced cooked turkey breast
> 1 (10¾-ounce) can Healthy Request Cream of Chicken Soup
> 1 cup chunky salsa (mild, medium, or hot)
> ½ cup (one 2.5-ounce jar) sliced mushrooms, drained
> 1 teaspoon dried parsley flakes
> ¼ teaspoon black pepper
> ⅓ cup Land O Lakes no-fat sour cream
> 3 cups hot cooked noodles, rinsed and drained

In a large skillet, combine turkey, chicken soup, salsa, mush-rooms, parsley flakes, and black pepper. Cook over medium heat for 5 minutes, or until mixture is heated through, stirring often. Add sour cream. Mix gently to combine. Lower heat and simmer for 3 to 4 minutes, stirring occasionally. For each serving, place ½ cup noo-dles on a plate and spoon about ½ cup turkey mixture over top.

HINTS: 1. If you don't have leftovers, purchase a chunk of cooked turkey breast from your local deli.
2. 2⅔ cups uncooked noodles usually cooks to about 3 cups.

Each serving equals:

HE: 1⅓ Protein • 1 Bread • ½ Vegetable • ½ Slider • 3 Optional Calories

190 Calories • 2 gm Fat • 11 gm Protein • 32 gm Carbohydrate • 813 mg Sodium • 78 mg Calcium • 1 gm Fiber

DIABETIC: 2 Starch • 1 Meat

Turkey 'n' Stuffing Casserole ❄

Everyone expects turkey and stuffing during the holidays, but can you imagine the looks of delight on your family's faces when you serve this savory dish in the middle of a March snowstorm?

◑ Serves 6

> 2 cups (one 16-ounce can) Healthy Request Chicken Broth
> 1 cup frozen peas
> 3 full cups (4½ ounces) dried bread cubes
> 1 teaspoon poultry seasoning
> 2 teaspoons dried onion flakes
> 1 teaspoon dried parsley flakes
> 1½ cups (8 ounces) diced cooked turkey breast
> 2 cups (one 16-ounce can) diced carrots, rinsed and drained

Preheat oven to 350 degrees. Spray an 8-by-8-inch baking dish with butter-flavored cooking spray. In a large saucepan, bring chicken broth to a boil. Stir in peas. Remove from heat. Add bread cubes, poultry seasoning, onion flakes, and parsley flakes. Mix well to combine. Stir in turkey and carrots. Pour mixture into prepared baking dish. Bake for 25 to 30 minutes. Place baking dish on a wire rack and let set for 5 minutes. Divide into 6 servings.

HINTS: 1. If you don't have leftovers, purchase a chunk of cooked turkey breast from your local deli.
2. Brownberry dried bread cubes work great.

Each serving equals:

HE: 1⅓ Protein • 1⅓ Bread • ⅔ Vegetable • 5 Optional Calories

161 Calories • 1 gm Fat • 12 gm Protein • 26 gm Carbohydrate • 879 mg Sodium • 22 mg Calcium • 3 gm Fiber

DIABETIC: 1 Meat • 1 Starch • 1 Vegetable

East Meets West Stir-Fry Skillet ❄

Stir-frying is a cooking technique we learned from Asian cuisine, but the ingredients in this stovetop dish are 100 percent all-American! Another "trick" we picked up from Eastern chefs—making a modest amount of meat and an abundance of vegetables into a perfectly satisfying meal. ♥ Serves 4

8 ounces ground 90% lean turkey or beef
½ teaspoon poultry seasoning
¼ teaspoon ground sage
¼ teaspoon garlic powder
4 cups purchased stir-fry vegetables
1 (10¾-ounce) can Healthy Request Tomato Soup
¼ teaspoon black pepper
2 cups hot cooked noodles, rinsed and drained

In a large skillet sprayed with butter-flavored cooking spray, brown meat. Stir in poultry seasoning, ground sage, and garlic powder. Add stir-fry vegetables. Mix well to combine. Lower heat and simmer for 8 to 10 minutes, stirring occasionally. Add tomato soup and black pepper. Mix well to combine. Continue simmering for 2 to 3 minutes. For each serving, place ½ cup noodles on a plate and top with scant 1 cup vegetable mixture.

HINTS: 1. 1¾ cups uncooked noodles usually cooks to about 2 cups.
2. Any combination of your choice of raw vegetables may be used in place of purchased stir-fry vegetables.

Each serving equals:

HE: 2 Vegetable • 1½ Protein • 1 Bread • ½ Slider • 5 Optional Calories

323 Calories • 7 gm Fat • 19 gm Protein •
46 gm Carbohydrate • 1501 mg Sodium •
120 mg Calcium • 6 gm Fiber

DIABETIC: 2 Vegetable • 2 Starch • 1½ Meat

Cheeseburger Noodle Skillet

I e-mailed my daughter-in-law Angie when this recipe was finally tested to my satisfaction. You see, when it comes to taste-testing anything "cheeseburger," my son Tommy usually gets the last word. His review: "Good enough to come home for!"

🌙 Serves 4 (1 cup)

> 8 ounces ground 90% lean turkey or beef
> ½ cup chopped onion
> 1¾ cups (one 15-ounce can) Hunt's Tomato Sauce
> 1 tablespoon Brown Sugar Twin
> ½ cup dill pickle relish
> ¼ teaspoon black pepper
> 2 cups hot cooked noodles, rinsed and drained
> ¾ cup (3 ounces) shredded Kraft reduced-fat Cheddar cheese

In a large skillet sprayed with butter-flavored cooking spray, brown meat and onion. Stir in tomato sauce, Brown Sugar Twin, pickle relish, and black pepper. Add noodles and Cheddar cheese. Mix well to combine. Lower heat and simmer for 10 minutes or until cheese melts, stirring occasionally.

HINT: 1¾ cups uncooked noodles usually cooks to about 2 cups.

Each serving equals:

HE: 2½ Protein • 2¼ Vegetable • 1 Bread •
1 Optional Calorie

---

281 Calories • 9 gm Fat • 21 gm Protein •
29 gm Carbohydrate • 1,339 mg Sodium •
204 mg Calcium • 3 gm Fiber

DIABETIC: 2 Meat • 2 Vegetable • 1 Starch

Squaw Corn Casserole ❄

It's such an all-American food, and it's the heart of what's best about Iowa. When you combine corn and ground meat with bread crumbs and spices, you've got a dish that would surely have made peace between the Indians and the pioneers! ☯ Serves 4

8 ounces ground 90% lean turkey or beef
2 cups (one 16-ounce can) whole-kernel corn, rinsed and drained
1 egg, beaten, or equivalent in egg substitute
⅓ cup water
⅓ cup Carnation Nonfat Dry Milk Powder
½ cup chopped onion
1½ teaspoons taco seasoning
¼ teaspoon black pepper
1 teaspoon dried parsley flakes
2 slices reduced-calorie white bread, made into crumbs

Preheat oven to 350 degrees. Spray an 8-by-8-inch baking dish with butter-flavored cooking spray. In a large skillet sprayed with butter-flavored cooking spray, brown meat. Remove from heat. In a large bowl, combine corn, egg, water, and dry milk powder. Stir in onion, taco seasoning, black pepper, and parsley flakes. Add browned meat and bread crumbs. Mix well to combine. Spread mixture into prepared baking dish. Bake for 40 to 45 minutes. Place baking dish on a wire rack and let set for 5 minutes. Divide into 4 servings.

Each serving equals:

HE: 1¾ Protein (¼ limited) • 1¼ Bread •
¼ Skim Milk • ¼ Vegetable

---

226 Calories • 6 gm Fat • 17 gm Protein •
26 gm Carbohydrate • 163 mg Sodium •
92 mg Calcium • 4 gm Fiber

DIABETIC: 2 Meat • 1½ Starch

Vegetable Meat Pie

So many favorite veggies in one dish make this easy meat pie a delectable winner in every household! It's also a great way to make a pound of meat feed a family of six—and believe me, no one will leave the table hungry. ☻ Serves 6

16 ounces ground 90% lean turkey or beef
½ cup finely chopped onion
¾ cup (1½ ounces) crushed Corn Chex
1½ teaspoons chili seasoning
1¾ cups (one 15-ounce can) Hunt's Tomato Sauce ☆
1 cup (one 8-ounce can) French-style green beans, rinsed and
*   drained*
1 cup (one 8-ounce can) diced carrots, rinsed and drained
½ cup frozen peas, thawed
½ cup frozen whole-kernel corn, thawed
1 tablespoon Brown Sugar Twin
1 teaspoon dried parsley flakes
1 teaspoon dried onion flakes

Preheat oven to 350 degrees. Spray a deep-dish 9-inch pie plate with olive oil–flavored cooking spray. In a large bowl, combine meat, onion, Corn Chex, chili seasoning, and ½ cup tomato sauce. Add green beans, carrots, peas, and corn. Mix well to combine. Pat mixture into prepared pie plate. Bake for 30 minutes. In a small bowl, combine remaining 1¼ cups tomato sauce, Brown Sugar Twin, parsley flakes, and onion flakes. Spread mixture evenly over meat mixture. Continue baking for 30 to 35 minutes. Place pie plate on a wire rack and let set for 5 minutes. Divide into 6 servings.

HINTS: 1. If you can't find diced carrots, use sliced carrots and coarsely chop.
2. Thaw peas and corn by placing in a colander and rinsing under hot water for one minute.

Each serving equals:

HE: 2 Protein • 2 Vegetable • ⅔ Bread • 1 Optional Calorie

---

178 Calories • 6 gm Fat • 16 gm Protein • 15 gm Carbohydrate • 584 mg Sodium • 20 mg Calcium • 3 gm Fiber

---

DIABETIC: 2 Meat • 2 Vegetable • ½ Starch

Sauerbraten Meatballs

My Bohemian ancestors should be smiling somewhere about this saucy, savory blend of meat and sauerkraut! It's a lovely dish for a family reunion, especially because the meatballs can easily be reheated and kept warm on a buffet table. ☻ Serves 6

16 ounces ground 90% lean turkey or beef

¾ cup finely chopped onion

⅔ cup (1½ ounces) instant potato flakes

¼ teaspoon black pepper

1¾ cups (one 15-ounce can) Hunt's Tomato Sauce ☆

1¾ cups (one 14½-ounce can) Bavarian-style sauerkraut, drained

½ teaspoon pumpkin pie spice

2 tablespoons Brown Sugar Twin

In a large bowl, combine meat, onion, potato flakes, black pepper, and ¼ cup tomato sauce. Mix well. Form into 24 (1-inch) meatballs. Place meatballs in an 8-by-12-inch glass baking dish. Cover and microwave on HIGH (100% power) for 3 minutes. Rearrange meatballs by moving outside pieces into center. Continue microwaving on HIGH for 4 to 5 minutes. Remove meatballs from baking dish and drain dish if necessary. Place sauerkraut in baking dish. Arrange meatballs over sauerkraut. In a small bowl, combine remaining 1½ cups tomato sauce, pumpkin pie spice, and Brown Sugar Twin. Spoon sauce mixture evenly over meatballs. Microwave on BAKE (80% power) for 4 to 6 minutes or until heated through. For each serving, place 4 meatballs on a plate and evenly spoon sauerkraut mixture over top.

HINT: Regular sauerkraut, ½ teaspoon caraway seeds, and 1 teaspoon Brown Sugar Twin may be substituted for Bavarian sauerkraut.

Each serving equals:

HE: 2 Protein • 2 Vegetable • ⅓ Bread •
2 Optional Calories

162 Calories • 6 gm Fat • 15 gm Protein •
12 gm Carbohydrate • 998 mg Sodium •
27 mg Calcium • 4 gm Fiber

DIABETIC: 2 Meat • 2 Vegetable

Momma's Porcupine Meatballs ❄

I'm not sure who first named these old-timey treats—probably a clever child who couldn't resist the comparison between these "spiky" rice-studded meatballs and that prickly little creature they resembled! Whatever you call them, your family will dine with delight. ☻ Serves 6

> 16 ounces ground 90% lean turkey or beef
> 1 cup (3 ounces) uncooked Minute Rice
> ¼ cup finely chopped onion
> 1 (10¾-ounce) can Healthy Request Tomato Soup ☆
> ¾ cup Healthy Request tomato juice or any reduced-sodium
>   tomato juice
> ¼ teaspoon dried minced garlic
> 1 teaspoon prepared mustard

In a large bowl, combine meat, uncooked rice, onion, and ¼ cup tomato soup. Form into 24 (1-inch) meatballs. Place meatballs in a large skillet sprayed with butter-flavored cooking spray, and brown meatballs for 3 to 4 minutes. Meanwhile, in a medium bowl, combine remaining tomato soup, tomato juice, garlic, and mustard. Pour mixture evenly over meatballs. Lower heat, cover, and simmer for 20 minutes, stirring occasionally. For each serving, place 4 meatballs on a plate and spoon about 3 tablespoons sauce over top.

Each serving equals:

HE: 2 Protein • ½ Bread • ⅓ Vegetable • ¼ Slider • 10 Optional Calories

179 Calories • 7 gm Fat • 15 gm Protein • 14 gm Carbohydrate • 254 mg Sodium • 12 mg Calcium • 1 gm Fiber

DIABETIC: 2 Meat • 1 Starch

Spinach Meatloaf

If you're having trouble getting your family to eat their veggies, you might want to try this fresh take on meatloaf that blends healthy chopped spinach into the mix—and tastes like the best kind of home cooking! The cheesy topping is pretty irresistible, too.

● Serves 6

16 ounces ground 90% lean turkey or beef
1 (10-ounce) package frozen chopped spinach, thawed and
  thoroughly drained
6 tablespoons (1½ ounces) dried fine bread crumbs
2 teaspoons Italian seasoning ☆
1¾ cups (one 15-ounce can) Hunt's Tomato Sauce ☆
2 teaspoons Sugar Twin or Sprinkle Sweet
¾ cup (3 ounces) shredded Kraft reduced-fat mozzarella cheese

Preheat oven to 350 degrees. Spray an 8-by-8-inch baking dish with butter-flavored cooking spray. In a large bowl, combine meat, spinach, bread crumbs, 1 teaspoon Italian seasoning, and ¼ cup tomato sauce. Mix well to combine. Pat mixture into prepared baking dish. Bake for 30 to 35 minutes. In a medium bowl, combine remaining 1½ cups tomato sauce, remaining 1 teaspoon Italian seasoning, sugar substitute, and mozzarella cheese. Spoon sauce mixture evenly over meatloaf. Continue baking for 15 to 20 minutes. Place baking dish on a wire rack and let set for 5 minutes. Cut into 6 servings.

Each serving equals:

HE: 2⅔ Protein • 1⅔ Vegetable • ⅓ Bread • 1 Optional Calorie

---

201 Calories • 9 gm Fat • 20 gm Protein • 10 gm Carbohydrate • 731 mg Sodium • 170 mg Calcium • 3 gm Fiber

---

DIABETIC: 2½ Meat • 2 Vegetable

Barbecue Burgers

Long for that tangy burst of barbecue flavor, but there's snow on the ground and the grill's in the garage? Never fear—I've got the answer in my healthy homemade barbecue sauce that turns your basic burger into irresistible fare. Be sure to allow enough time for the sauce's ingredients to get truly "up close and personal"!

☻ Serves 8

16 ounces ground 90% lean turkey or beef
1 cup finely chopped onion
1 cup finely chopped celery
1 cup chopped fresh mushrooms
1 cup Healthy Request tomato juice or any reduced-sodium
 tomato juice
¼ cup Heinz Light Harvest Ketchup or any reduced-sodium ketchup
2 teaspoons chili seasoning
¼ teaspoon black pepper
2 tablespoons Quick Cooking Minute Tapioca
8 reduced-calorie hamburger buns

In a large skillet sprayed with olive oil–flavored cooking spray, brown meat, onion, celery, and mushrooms. Add tomato juice, ketchup, chili seasoning, and black pepper. Mix well to combine. Lower heat and simmer for 10 minutes. Stir in tapioca. Continue simmering for 3 to 4 minutes, stirring occasionally. For each sandwich, spoon about ½ cup meat mixture between 2 halves of a bun.

Each serving equals:

HE: 1½ Protein • 1 Bread • 1 Vegetable •
13 Optional Calories

198 Calories • 6 gm Fat • 13 gm Protein •
23 gm Carbohydrate • 329 mg Sodium •
19 mg Calcium • 1 gm Fiber

DIABETIC: 1½ Meat • 1 Starch • 1 Vegetable

Iowa Farm Boy Reubens

This classic deli sandwich is widely beloved but oh-so-high in fat and calories that most people have eliminated it from their healthy lifestyle menus. Now you don't have to anymore—when you prepare this dish using some of the best fat-free and reduced-fat products. It's true what they say: You can't keep 'em down on the farm anymore. This kind of good news gets out!   ☻   Serves 6

    16 ounces ground 90% lean turkey or beef
    ¼ teaspoon black pepper
    ¼ teaspoon ground sage
    ¼ teaspoon garlic powder
    ¼ teaspoon poultry seasoning
    1 cup (one 8-ounce can) sauerkraut, well drained
    2 tablespoons Kraft Fat Free Thousand Island Dressing
    6 reduced-calorie hamburger buns
    6 (¾-ounce) slices Kraft reduced-fat Swiss cheese
    1 (medium-sized) tomato, cut into 6 slices

In a large bowl, combine meat, black pepper, sage, garlic powder, and poultry seasoning. Using scant ⅓ cup as measure, form into 6 patties. Place patties in a large skillet sprayed with butter-flavored cooking spray. Brown patties for about 5 minutes on each side. Meanwhile, in a small saucepan, combine well-drained sauerkraut and Thousand Island dressing. Cook over medium heat until heated through. For each sandwich, place a browned patty on the bottom half of a bun, top with 2 full tablespoons sauerkraut mixture, arrange 1 slice Swiss cheese and 1 slice tomato over top, and cover with top half of bun.

Each serving equals:

    HE: 3 Protein • 1 Bread • ½ Vegetable •
    8 Optional Calories
    _____
    236 Calories • 8 gm Fat • 22 gm Protein •
    19 gm Carbohydrate • 595 mg Sodium •
    221 mg Calcium • 2 gm Fiber
    _____
    DIABETIC: 3 Meat • 1 Starch • ½ Vegetable

Pam's Meatza Pie

My daughter-in-law Pam is a wonderful cook with a passion for all things Italian, so this dish was created with her taste buds in mind! Are you surprised to find cottage cheese in this inventive concoction? Just wait till you see the magic it works when combined with the Parmesan and mozzarella cheeses!   ☻   Serves 6

> *8 ounces ground 90% lean turkey or beef*
> *½ cup chopped onion*
> *1 cup (one 8-ounce can) Hunt's Tomato Sauce*
> *½ cup (one 2.5-ounce jar) sliced mushrooms, drained*
> *2 teaspoons Italian seasoning*
> *2 cups hot cooked noodles, rinsed and drained*
> *1½ cups fat-free cottage cheese*
> *¼ cup (¾ ounce) grated Kraft fat-free Parmesan cheese*
> *2 cups (one 16-ounce can) French-style green beans, rinsed and*
>   *drained*
> *¾ cup (3 ounces) shredded Kraft reduced-fat mozzarella*
>   *cheese*

Preheat oven to 375 degrees. Spray a deep-dish 9-inch pie plate with olive oil–flavored cooking spray. In a large skillet sprayed with olive oil–flavored cooking spray, brown meat and onion. Stir in tomato sauce, mushrooms, and Italian seasoning. Spread noodles into prepared pie plate. Spoon meat mixture over noodles. In a medium bowl, combine cottage cheese and Parmesan cheese. Stir in green beans. Spoon cottage cheese mixture evenly over meat mixture. Sprinkle mozzarella cheese evenly over top. Bake for 35 to 40 minutes. Place pie plate on a wire rack and let set for 5 minutes. Cut into 6 wedges.

HINT: 1¾ cups uncooked noodles usually cooks to about 2 cups.

Each serving equals:

HE: 2⅓ Protein • 1⅔ Vegetable • ⅔ Bread

242 Calories • 6 gm Fat • 23 gm Protein •
24 gm Carbohydrate • 753 mg Sodium •
150 mg Calcium • 3 gm Fiber

DIABETIC: 2 Meat • 2 Vegetable • 1 Starch

Micro Stroganoff

Did you know that microwaving even lean meat is a great way to save on fat without sacrificing flavor? This creamy, Russian-inspired classic stirs up some real magic without costing you excess calories. Best of all, you're rewarded for your healthy lifestyle choices by dining on something splendid!   ☻   Serves 4

> 8 ounces ground 90% lean turkey or beef
> 2 teaspoons dried onion flakes
> 1 (10¾-ounce) can Healthy Request Cream of Mushroom Soup
> ⅓ cup Carnation Nonfat Dry Milk Powder
> ¾ cup water
> ½ cup (one 2.5-ounce jar) sliced mushrooms, drained
> 1 teaspoon Worcestershire sauce
> ½ teaspoon dried minced garlic
> ¼ teaspoon black pepper
> ¾ cup Yoplait plain fat-free yogurt
> 1 teaspoon cornstarch
> 2 cups hot cooked noodles, rinsed and drained

Crumble meat into a plastic colander and set colander in a glass pie plate. Microwave on HIGH (100% power) for 5 minutes, stirring after 2 minutes to break apart. Set aside. In an 8-cup glass measuring bowl, combine onion flakes, mushroom soup, dry milk powder, and water. Stir in mushrooms, Worcestershire sauce, garlic, and black pepper. Add browned meat. Mix well to combine. Cover and microwave on HIGH for 5 to 6 minutes or until hot and bubbly. In a small bowl, combine yogurt and cornstarch. Stir yogurt mixture into meat mixture. Re-cover and microwave on HIGH for 1 minute or until heated through. For each serving, place ½ cup noodles on a plate and spoon about ⅔ cup meat mixture over top.

HINT: 1¾ cups uncooked noodles usually cooks to about 2 cups.

Each serving equals:

HE: 1½ Protein • 1 Bread • ½ Skim Milk •
¼ Vegetable • ½ Slider • 4 Optional Calories

279 Calories • 7 gm Fat • 19 gm Protein •
35 gm Carbohydrate • 519 mg Sodium •
220 mg Calcium • 2 gm Fiber

DIABETIC: 2 Starch • 1½ Meat • ½ Skim Milk

Mexican Pot Pie

Remember how Grandma used to serve her old-fashioned pot pies with a biscuit topping? Mmm-hmm! Well, memories are terrific, but isn't it better to bring back that great taste in this delightful South of the Border entree that makes every meal a fiesta?

● Serves 6

> 8 ounces ground 90% lean turkey or beef
> ½ cup chopped onion
> ¾ cup frozen whole-kernel corn, thawed
> 10 ounces (one 16-ounce can) kidney beans, rinsed and
>   drained
> 1 (10¾-ounce) can Healthy Request Tomato Soup
> ½ cup chunky salsa (mild, medium, or hot)
> 1 teaspoon chili seasoning
> ¾ cup (3 ounces) shredded Kraft reduced-fat Cheddar cheese
> 1 (7.5-ounce) can Pillsbury refrigerated buttermilk biscuits

Preheat oven to 400 degrees. Spray an 8-by-8-inch baking dish with olive oil–flavored cooking spray. In a large skillet sprayed with olive oil–flavored cooking spray, brown meat and onion. Stir in corn, kidney beans, tomato soup, salsa, chili seasoning, and Cheddar cheese. Lower heat and simmer for 5 minutes, stirring occasionally. Pour mixture into prepared baking dish. Separate biscuits and cut each into 3 pieces. Evenly sprinkle biscuit pieces over meat mixture. Lightly spray biscuit tops with olive oil–flavored cooking spray. Bake for 12 to 15 minutes or until biscuits are golden brown. Place baking dish on a wire rack and let set for 5 minutes. Divide into 6 servings.

HINT: Thaw corn by placing in a colander and rinsing under hot water for one minute.

Each serving equals:

HE: 2½ Protein • 1½ Bread • ⅓ Vegetable •
¼ Slider • 10 Optional Calories

---

279 Calories • 7 gm Fat • 17 gm Protein •
37 gm Carbohydrate • 698 mg Sodium •
148 mg Calcium • 6 gm Fiber

DIABETIC: 2½ Starch • 2 Meat

Sausage Carrot Supper

Do you find it hard to believe that plain old ground meat, blended with a few spices, can actually fool your taste buds into thinking they're enjoying real sausage? The proof is in the eating—and this delicious baked casserole will surprise and delight you with its tangy flavors. Ya gotta believe! ● Serves 4

8 ounces ground 90% lean
    turkey or beef
½ teaspoon poultry seasoning
¼ teaspoon ground sage
¼ teaspoon garlic powder
½ cup diced celery
½ cup chopped onion
1½ cups shredded carrots

1½ cups cooked rice
¾ cup (3 ounces) shredded
    Kraft reduced-fat
    Cheddar cheese
1 (10¾-ounce) can Healthy
    Request Tomato Soup
¼ teaspoon black pepper
⅓ cup water

Preheat oven to 350 degrees. Spray an 8-by-8-inch baking dish with butter-flavored cooking spray. In a large skillet sprayed with butter-flavored cooking spray, brown meat with poultry seasoning, sage, garlic powder, celery, onion, and carrots. Add rice, Cheddar cheese, tomato soup, black pepper, and water. Mix well to combine. Pour mixture into prepared baking dish. Bake for 30 minutes. Place baking dish on a wire rack and let set for 5 minutes. Divide into 4 servings.

HINT: 1 cup uncooked rice usually cooks to about 1½ cups.

Each serving equals:

HE: 2½ Protein • 1¼ Vegetable • ¾ Bread •
½ Slider • 5 Optional Calories

277 Calories • 9 gm Fat • 19 gm Protein •
30 gm Carbohydrate • 508 mg Sodium •
190 mg Calcium • 2 gm Fiber

DIABETIC: 2 Meat • 1½ Starch • 1 Vegetable

Hawaiian JOs

Even if Hawaii is a long, long, long way from where you live, you and your family can enjoy a lip-smacking taste of the tropics tonight with this variation on traditional Sloppy Joes. You could also serve this fruited combination over rice, and you'll find that leftovers reheat beautifully. ☺ Serves 8

16 ounces ground 90% lean turkey or beef
½ cup chopped onion
½ cup chopped green bell pepper
1 teaspoon dried minced garlic
1 cup (one 8-ounce can) Hunt's Tomato Sauce
1 teaspoon Worcestershire sauce
2 tablespoons Brown Sugar Twin
1 teaspoon prepared mustard
1 cup (one 8-ounce can) crushed pineapple, packed in fruit juice, undrained
8 reduced-calorie hamburger buns

In a large skillet sprayed with butter-flavored cooking spray, brown meat, onion, green pepper, and garlic. Stir in tomato sauce, Worcestershire sauce, Brown Sugar Twin, and mustard. Lower heat and simmer for 5 minutes. Add undrained pineapple. Mix well to combine. Continue simmering for 10 minutes, stirring occasionally. For each sandwich, spoon a full ⅓ cup meat mixture between 2 halves of a bun.

Each serving equals:

HE: 1½ Protein • 1 Bread • ¾ Vegetable • ¼ Fruit • 1 Optional Calorie

190 Calories • 6 gm Fat • 12 gm Protein •
22 gm Carbohydrate • 429 mg Sodium •
11 mg Calcium • 2 gm Fiber

DIABETIC: 1½ Meat • 1 Starch • 1 Vegetable

Creamy Beef 'n' Noodles

Remember how "diet" food used to taste—dry, flavorless, or bland? Well, now that cooking healthy is your goal, you never have to settle for that awful stuff again! Nothing could be more convincing than this scrumptious baked-noodle entree that practically "oozes" creamy goodness! (My own "meat and potatoes" guy doesn't mind if I limit his meat as long as I "beef" up the flavor!)

◑ Serves 6

> ¾ cup diced onion
> 1¾ cups (one 14½-ounce can) Swanson Beef Broth
> 1¾ cups (3 ounces) uncooked noodles
> 2 cups (12 ounces) cubed cooked lean roast beef
> 1 cup frozen whole-kernel corn, thawed
> 2 tablespoons all-purpose flour
> ⅔ cup Carnation Nonfat Dry Milk Powder
> ¾ cup water
> ⅛ teaspoon black pepper
> 1 teaspoon dried parsley flakes

Preheat oven to 350 degrees. Spray an 8-by-8-inch baking dish with butter-flavored cooking spray. In a large saucepan, cook onion in beef broth for 5 minutes. Add uncooked noodles, roast beef, and corn. Mix well to combine. Bring mixture to a boil. Lower heat and simmer for 6 to 8 minutes or until noodles are tender, stirring occasionally. In a covered jar, combine flour, dry milk powder, and water. Shake well to blend. Pour milk mixture into noodle mixture. Mix well to combine. Stir in black pepper and parsley flakes. Continue simmering until sauce thickens, stirring often. Pour mixture into prepared baking dish. Bake for 25 to 30 minutes. Place baking dish on a wire rack and let set for 5 minutes. Divide into 6 servings.

HINTS: 1. If you don't have leftovers, purchase a chunk of cooked roast beef from your local deli.
2. Thaw corn by placing in a colander and rinsing under hot water for one minute.

Each serving equals:

HE: 2 Protein • 1 Bread • ¼ Skim Milk •
¼ Vegetable • 15 Optional Calories

---

245 Calories • 5 gm Fat • 23 gm Protein •
27 gm Carbohydrate • 323 mg Sodium •
107 mg Calcium • 2 gm Fiber

DIABETIC: 2 Meat • 1½ Starch

Creamy "Pot Roast" Skillet

When you don't want to "heat up" the kitchen by turning on the stove, a skillet supper is a great idea. This meaty noodle dish requires only a little watching and stirring before it's ready to serve up to your hungry troops. Now, wasn't that easy?

☻ Serves 4 (1¼ cups)

> 8 ounces ground 90% lean turkey or beef
> ½ cup chopped onion
> 1¾ cups (one 14½-ounce can) Swanson Beef Broth
> 1¾ cups (3 ounces) uncooked noodles
> 1½ cups frozen cut green beans, thawed
> 1½ cups frozen sliced carrots, thawed
> 1 (10¾-ounce) can Healthy Request Cream of Mushroom Soup
> ¼ teaspoon black pepper
> 1 teaspoon dried parsley flakes

In a large skillet sprayed with butter-flavored cooking spray, brown meat and onion. Add beef broth. Mix well to combine. Stir in uncooked noodles, green beans, and carrots. Bring mixture to a boil. Lower heat, cover, and simmer for 15 minutes or until noodles and vegetables are tender, stirring occasionally. Stir in mushroom soup, black pepper, and parsley flakes. Continue simmering for 15 minutes or until mixture is heated through, stirring occasionally.

HINTS: 1. Thaw green beans and carrots by placing in a colander and rinsing under hot water for one minute.
2. 1 full cup (6 ounces) diced lean cooked roast beef may be used in place of ground meat.

Each serving equals:

HE: 1¾ Vegetable • 1½ Protein • 1 Bread • ½ Slider • 10 Optional Calories

---

264 Calories • 8 gm Fat • 16 gm Protein • 32 gm Carbohydrate • 743 mg Sodium • 94 mg Calcium • 4 gm Fiber

---

DIABETIC: 1½ Vegetable • 1½ Meat • 1½ Starch

Cozy Crock Comfort

If you haven't yet dug your Crock-Pot out of the attic, I bet this recipe will make you do it today! It's a perfect slow-cooked dish, ready to serve in minutes after the busiest day, and it's especially handy if your family doesn't always manage to sit down together at the table. This way, the food stays cozy-warm but doesn't get over-cooked. ☻ Serves 6 (1 full cup)

16 ounces ground 90% lean turkey or beef
½ cup chopped onion
3 cups (15 ounces) diced raw potatoes
⅓ cup (1 ounce) uncooked regular rice
1½ cups shredded carrots
1 cup finely diced celery
1½ cups Healthy Request tomato juice or any reduced-sodium
    tomato juice
1 (10¾-ounce) can Healthy Request Tomato Soup
¼ teaspoon black pepper
1 teaspoon dried parsley flakes

In a large skillet sprayed with butter-flavored cooking spray, brown meat. Place browned meat in a slow cooker container. Add onion, potatoes, uncooked rice, carrots, and celery. Mix well to combine. Stir in tomato juice, tomato soup, black pepper, and parsley flakes. Cover and cook on LOW for 6 to 8 hours. Mix well before serving.

Each serving equals:

HE: 2 Protein • 1½ Vegetable • ⅔ Bread • ¼ Slider • 10 Optional Calories

243 Calories • 7 gm Fat • 16 gm Protein • 29 gm Carbohydrate • 290 mg Sodium • 33 mg Calcium • 3 gm Fiber

DIABETIC: 2 Meat • 1½ Starch • 1 Vegetable

Chunky Stew with Biscuits

I get a lot of requests for microwave main dishes from busy moms who are tired of serving frozen dinners all the time but who aren't sure how else to cook in the microwave. This delectable stew is nourishing and tasty but wonderfully simple to serve up fast. It's great made from leftover meat, but you can also purchase a chunk of deli roast beef on your way home.   ☻   Serves 6

> *1 cup finely chopped celery*
> *1½ cups sliced carrots*
> *½ cup chopped onion*
> *¼ cup water*
> *1½ cups (8 ounces) diced cooked lean roast beef*
> *½ cup frozen peas, thawed*
> *1 (12-ounce) jar Heinz Fat-Free Beef Gravy*
> *1½ tablespoons dried fine bread crumbs*
> *1 teaspoon dried parsley flakes*
> *½ teaspoon paprika*
> *1 (7.5-ounce) can Pillsbury refrigerated buttermilk biscuits*

Place celery, carrots, onion, and water in an 8-by-8-inch glass baking dish. Cover and microwave on HIGH (100% power) for 6 to 8 minutes or until vegetables are tender. Stir in roast beef, peas, and gravy. Re-cover and microwave on HIGH for 3 to 4 minutes. Mix well to combine. Place bread crumbs, parsley flakes, and paprika in a small bowl. Separate biscuits and cut each into 3 pieces. Place biscuit pieces on top of stew mixture. Lightly spray biscuit tops with butter-flavored cooking spray. Sprinkle bread crumb mixture evenly over biscuits. Microwave on HIGH, uncovered, for 3 to 4 minutes or until biscuits spring back when lightly touched. Place baking dish on a wire rack and let set for 5 minutes. Divide into 6 servings.

HINT: Thaw peas by placing in a colander and rinsing under hot water for one minute.

Each serving equals:

HE: 1½ Bread • 1⅓ Protein • 1 Vegetable •
¼ Slider • 5 Optional Calories

217 Calories • 5 gm Fat • 17 gm Protein •
26 gm Carbohydrate • 693 mg Sodium •
33 mg Calcium • 4 gm Fiber

DIABETIC: 1½ Starch • 1 Meat • 1 Vegetable

Cliff's Calico Skillet

If your goal is to get your family to eat lots more fiber, here's a smart way to do it in no time at all! It's ready so quickly, you'll probably serve this skillet supper often—which I know will make Cliff very proud, since he inspired it. ☺ Serves 4 (1 cup)

> 8 ounces ground 90% lean turkey or beef
> ½ cup chopped onion
> 1 cup frozen whole-kernel corn, thawed
> 10 ounces (one 16-ounce can) great northern beans, rinsed and
>   drained
> 2 cups (one 16-ounce can) cut green beans, rinsed and drained
> 1 (10¾-ounce) can Healthy Request Tomato Soup
> 1 teaspoon taco seasoning
> 1 teaspoon dried parsley flakes
> ¼ teaspoon black pepper

In a large skillet sprayed with olive oil–flavored cooking spray, brown meat and onion. Stir in corn, great northern beans, green beans, and tomato soup. Add taco seasoning, parsley flakes, and black pepper. Mix well to combine. Lower heat and simmer for 5 to 6 minutes, stirring occasionally.

HINT: Thaw corn by placing in a colander and rinsing under hot water for one minute.

Each serving equals:

HE: 2¾ Protein • 1¼ Vegetable • ½ Bread •
½ Slider • 5 Optional Calories

---

278 Calories • 6 gm Fat • 19 gm Protein •
37 gm Carbohydrate • 289 mg Sodium •
80 mg Calcium • 7 gm Fiber

DIABETIC: 2 Meat • 2 Starch • 1 Vegetable

Palisades Pork

✻

I named this dish after the famous amusement park on New Jersey's Palisades, where fun was the name of the game! This dish provides so much culinary pleasure, your taste buds will think they're riding a roller coaster of terrific tastes worthy of a few screams of joy, but try to control yourself—the neighbors are sure to be jealous!

◐ Serves 4

> 2 tablespoons Kraft Fat Free Italian Dressing
> 4 (4-ounce) tenderized lean pork tenderloins
> 1¾ cups (one 15-ounce can) Hunt's Tomato Sauce
> 1 tablespoon all-purpose flour
> 1 teaspoon Italian seasoning
> 2 teaspoons Sugar Twin or Sprinkle Sweet
> ¼ cup (1 ounce) sliced ripe olives
> ½ cup (one 2.5-ounce jar) sliced mushrooms, drained
> ¼ teaspoon black pepper
> ¼ cup (¾ ounce) grated Kraft fat-free Parmesan cheese

Pour Italian dressing into a large skillet. Place meat in skillet. Cook over medium heat, browning meat on both sides. In a medium bowl, combine tomato sauce, flour, Italian seasoning, sugar substitute, olives, mushrooms, and black pepper. Pour mixture over meat. Lower heat, cover, and simmer for 10 minutes, stirring occasionally. For each serving, place 1 piece of meat on a plate, spoon ½ cup sauce over meat, and sprinkle 1 tablespoon Parmesan cheese over top.

HINT: Don't overbrown meat or it will become tough.

Each serving equals:

> HE: 3¼ Protein • 2 Vegetable • ¼ Fat •
> 9 Optional Calories
>
> ---
>
> 227 Calories • 7 gm Fat • 27 gm Protein •
> 14 gm Carbohydrate • 1,122 mg Sodium •
> 34 mg Calcium • 3 gm Fiber
>
> ---
>
> DIABETIC: 3 Meat • 2 Vegetable

Asparagus-Egg-Ham Scallop

If you've never cooked with fresh asparagus, depending instead on the canned variety, I think you'll be very pleased by the delicious difference in taste and texture in this recipe! This creamy blend also delivers a healthy boost of calcium along with great flavor.

◑ Serves 4

> 2 cups cut fresh asparagus
> 1½ cups hot water
> 1½ cups (one 12-fluid-ounce can) Carnation Evaporated Skim Milk
> 3 tablespoons all-purpose flour
> ½ teaspoon lemon pepper
> ⅛ teaspoon paprika
> 2 hard-boiled eggs, sliced
> 1 full cup (6 ounces) diced Dubuque 97% fat-free ham or any extra-lean ham
> 1 teaspoon dried parsley flakes
> ⅓ cup (1½ ounces) shredded Kraft reduced-fat Cheddar cheese

Preheat oven to 350 degrees. Spray an 8-by-8-inch baking dish with butter-flavored cooking spray. In a medium saucepan, cook asparagus in water for 5 minutes or until tender. Drain. In a covered jar, combine evaporated skim milk and flour. Shake well to blend. Pour into a medium saucepan sprayed with butter-flavored cooking spray. Add lemon pepper and paprika. Mix well to combine. Cook over medium heat until mixture thickens and starts to boil, stirring often. Remove from heat. In a large bowl, combine eggs, asparagus, ham, and parsley flakes. Add sauce mixture. Mix gently to combine. Pour mixture into prepared baking dish. Evenly sprinkle Cheddar cheese over top. Bake for 15 minutes. Place baking dish on a wire rack and let set for 5 minutes. Divide into 4 servings.

HINT: If you want the look and feel of eggs without the cholesterol, toss out the yolks and dice the whites.

Each serving equals:

HE: 2 Protein (½ limited) • 1 Vegetable •
¾ Skim Milk • ¼ Bread

222 Calories • 6 gm Fat • 22 gm Protein •
20 gm Carbohydrate • 589 mg Sodium •
374 mg Calcium • 2 gm Fiber

DIABETIC: 2 Meat • 1 Vegetable • 1 Skim Milk

German Pork and Dressing ❄

Combining delicious lean pork with sweet 'n' tangy fruit is a wonderful European tradition I decided to bring back home in this recipe that's especially tasty on a crisp fall night! The veggies provide welcome amounts of fiber, but it's the crumbly dressing that makes this dish taste so special.   ☻   Serves 4

6 slices reduced-calorie bread, made into soft crumbs
½ cup (3 ounces) diced dried apricots
2 tablespoons raisins
1 cup finely chopped celery
1 cup shredded carrots
½ cup unsweetened apple juice
½ cup water
½ teaspoon apple pie spice
4 (4-ounce) lean pork tenderloins or cutlets

Preheat oven to 350 degrees. Spray an 8-by-8-inch baking dish with butter-flavored cooking spray. In a large bowl, combine bread crumbs, apricots, raisins, celery, and carrots. In a small bowl, combine apple juice, water, and apple pie spice. Add juice mixture to bread mixture. Mix well to combine. Pat mixture into prepared baking dish. In a large skillet sprayed with butter-flavored cooking spray, lightly brown meat on both sides. Place browned meat over dressing mixture. Cover and bake for 40 to 45 minutes. Uncover and continue baking for 10 to 15 minutes. Place baking dish on a wire rack and let set for 5 minutes. Divide into 4 servings.

Each serving equals:

HE: 3 Protein • 1½ Fruit • 1 Vegetable • ¾ Bread

278 Calories • 6 gm Fat • 29 gm Protein •
27 gm Carbohydrate • 285 mg Sodium •
77 mg Calcium • 5 gm Fiber

DIABETIC: 3 Meat • 1 Fruit • 1 Vegetable • 1 Starch

Ham and Broccoli Fettuccine

If you've only been using your microwave lately to reheat coffee and heat frozen dinners, why not add this tasty pasta dish to your repertoire? This couldn't be simpler or faster to prepare, and it delivers so much luscious flavor, you'll be certain to win applause when you carry this to the table. ☻ Serves 4 (1 cup)

1½ cups frozen cut broccoli, thawed
1 full cup (6 ounces) chopped Dubuque 97% fat-free ham or any extra-lean ham
2 cups hot cooked fettuccine or noodles, rinsed and drained
½ teaspoon lemon pepper
¼ cup (¾ ounce) grated Kraft fat-free Parmesan cheese
½ cup water
⅓ cup Carnation Nonfat Dry Milk Powder

In an 8-cup glass measuring bowl, combine broccoli and ham. Microwave on HIGH (100% power) for 4 minutes. Mix well to combine. Stir in fettuccine, lemon pepper, and Parmesan cheese. In a small bowl, combine water and dry milk powder. Add milk mixture to fettuccine mixture. Mix well to combine. Cover and microwave on HIGH for 2 minutes. Let set for 3 minutes. Mix gently before serving.

HINTS: 1. Thaw broccoli by placing in a colander and rinsing under hot water for one minute.
2. 1½ cups broken uncooked fettuccine usually cooks to about 2 cups.

Each serving equals:

HE: 1¼ Protein • 1 Bread • ¾ Vegetable •
¼ Skim Milk

194 Calories • 2 gm Fat • 14 gm Protein •
30 gm Carbohydrate • 513 mg Sodium •
90 mg Calcium • 3 gm Fiber

DIABETIC: 1½ Starch • 1 Meat • 1 Vegetable

Creamy Broccoli and Ham Bake ❄

Are you a non-cook cook, someone who usually looks at recipes and thinks, "Not me!" This dish is custom-made for people who insist they haven't got the time or inclination to cook healthy. What could be simpler? Five ingredients, heat 'em in a skillet, pour 'em in a dish, and bake, then eat. Maybe you really are a cook, after all!

☻ Serves 4

> 1 (10¾-ounce) can Healthy Request Cream of Broccoli or
>   Mushroom Soup
> 4 (¾-ounce) slices Kraft reduced-fat Swiss cheese, shredded
> 2 cups frozen chopped broccoli, thawed
> 2 cups hot cooked noodles, rinsed and drained
> 1 full cup (6 ounces) diced Dubuque 97% fat-free ham or any
>   extra-lean ham

Preheat oven to 350 degrees. Spray an 8-by-8-inch baking dish with butter-flavored cooking spray. In a large saucepan, combine broccoli soup, Swiss cheese, and broccoli. Cook over medium-low heat until cheese melts, stirring often. Stir in noodles and ham. Pour mixture into prepared baking dish. Bake for 25 to 30 minutes. Place baking dish on a wire rack and let set for 5 minutes. Divide into 4 servings.

HINTS: 1. Thaw broccoli by placing in a colander and rinsing under hot water for one minute.
   2. 1¾ cups uncooked noodles usually cooks to about 2 cups.

Each serving equals:

HE: 2 Protein • 1 Vegetable • 1 Bread • ½ Slider, 1 Optional Calorie

---

241 Calories • 5 gm Fat • 19 gm Protein, •
30 gm Carbohydrate • 733 mg Sodium •
285 mg Calcium • 2 gm Fiber

DIABETIC: 2 Meat • 1½ Starch • 1 Vegetable

Red Rice Skillet

This quick-fix recipe makes a satisfying summer lunch when the tomatoes in your garden are rosy red and oh-so-sweet! If you like your food just a bit spicier, you could add a spoonful or two of salsa to give this tasty dish even more sparkle.

◐ Serves 4 (1 cup)

½ cup chopped onion

1 full cup (6 ounces) finely diced Dubuque 97% fat-free ham or any extra-lean ham

2 cups peeled and chopped fresh tomatoes

1 cup Healthy Request tomato juice or any reduced-sodium tomato juice

1 tablespoon chopped fresh parsley or 1 teaspoon dried parsley flakes

1½ teaspoons taco seasoning

¼ teaspoon black pepper

1 cup (3 ounces) uncooked Minute Rice

1 tablespoon Brown Sugar Twin

In a large skillet sprayed with butter-flavored cooking spray, sauté onion and ham for 5 minutes or until lightly browned. Stir in tomatoes, tomato juice, parsley, taco seasoning, and black pepper. Bring mixture to a boil. Add uncooked rice and Brown Sugar Twin. Mix well to combine. Cover and remove from heat. Let set for 5 minutes. Fluff well with a fork before serving.

Each serving equals:

HE: 1¾ Vegetable • 1 Protein • ¾ Bread • 1 Optional Calorie

126 Calories • 2 gm Fat • 9 gm Protein • 18 gm Carbohydrate • 406 mg Sodium • 21 mg Calcium • 2 gm Fiber

DIABETIC: 1½ Vegetable • 1 Meat • 1 Starch

Nancy's Ham Rolls

Here's an unusual (and unusually delicious) way to serve ham, especially to young children. Rolled in a mouth-watering sauce, then in a "secret" ingredient (the graham cracker crumbs), these "balls" also make a wonderful choice for a party buffet. Thanks to our friend Nancy Wacker for starting the "idea" ball rolling!

◐ Serves 8 (2 each)

> 3 cups (16 ounces) ground Dubuque 97% fat-free ham or any
>   extra-lean ham
> 8 ounces ground 90% lean turkey or beef
> 1½ cups purchased graham cracker crumbs or 24 (2½-inch)
>   graham cracker squares made into fine crumbs
> ⅔ cup Carnation Nonfat Dry Milk Powder
> ½ cup water
> 1 (10¾-ounce) can Healthy Request Tomato Soup
> ¼ cup white vinegar
> ½ cup Sugar Twin or Sprinkle Sweet
> 2 tablespoons Brown Sugar Twin
> 1 teaspoon prepared mustard
> 1 tablespoon dried parsley flakes

Preheat oven to 350 degrees. Spray a 9-by-13-inch baking dish with butter-flavored cooking spray. In a large bowl, combine ground ham, ground meat, and graham cracker crumbs. In a small bowl, combine dry milk powder and water. Add milk mixture to meat mixture. Mix well to combine. Let set for 5 minutes. Using a ¼-cup measure as a guide, form into 16 balls. Place ham balls in prepared baking dish. In a medium bowl, combine tomato soup, vinegar, Sugar Twin, Brown Sugar Twin, mustard, and parsley flakes. Drizzle soup mixture evenly over ham balls. Bake for 45 to 50 minutes, basting occasionally with sauce.

HINTS: 1. Grind ham in a blender, if you don't have a grinder.
2. If you want, place 8 balls each in two 8-by-8-inch baking dishes, drizzle sauce evenly over top, and bake as usual, but freeze one of the dishes for future use.

Each serving equals:

HE: 2 Protein • 1 Bread • ¼ Skim Milk • ¼ Slider • 15 Optional Calories

239 Calories • 7 gm Fat • 18 gm Protein • 26 gm Carbohydrate • 797 mg Sodium • 82 mg Calcium • 1 gm Fiber

DIABETIC: 2 Meat • 1½ Starch

Potato Ham Bake

This dish takes a few minutes to assemble, but once it's in the oven, you can relax while it bakes to a wonderfully crusty and fragrant perfection. My grandsons are fans of this cozy dish and love picking out the little bits of ham among the potatoes!

○ Serves 6

4 cups (20 ounces) diced raw
    potatoes
1½ cups (9 ounces) diced
    Dubuque 97% fat-free
    ham or any extra-lean
    ham
¾ cup diced onion
⅔ cup Carnation Nonfat Dry
    Milk Powder

½ cup water
1 (10¾-ounce) can Healthy
    Request Cream of
    Mushroom Soup
1 teaspoon prepared mustard
1 teaspoon dried parsley flakes
¼ teaspoon black pepper
¼ teaspoon paprika

Preheat oven to 375 degrees. Spray an 8-by-8-inch baking dish with butter-flavored cooking spray. Layer half of potatoes, ham, and onion in prepared baking dish. Repeat layers, finishing with a potato layer. In a small bowl, combine dry milk powder, water, mushroom soup, mustard, parsley flakes, and black pepper. Pour mixture evenly over top of potato layer. Sprinkle paprika evenly over top. Cover and bake for 60 minutes. Uncover and continue baking for 15 minutes. Place baking dish on a wire rack and let set for 5 minutes. Divide into 6 servings.

Each serving equals:

HE: 1 Protein • ⅔ Bread • ⅓ Skim Milk •
¼ Vegetable • ¼ Slider • 8 Optional Calories

167 Calories • 3 gm Fat • 12 gm Protein •
23 gm Carbohydrate • 617 mg Sodium •
138 mg Calcium • 1 gm Fiber

DIABETIC: 1½ Starch • 1 Meat

Bavarian Stroganoff

Here's a truly luscious, Old-World-flavored main dish that will dazzle your guests with its "forbidden" flavors! Can anything this
scrumptious and soul-satisfying really be good for your heart? Yes,
yes, yes!   ❤   Serves 4 (1¼ cups)

> 1 full cup (6 ounces) finely diced Dubuque 97% fat-free ham or
>   any extra-lean ham
> ¼ cup finely diced onion
> 1 (10¾-ounce) can Healthy Request Cream of Mushroom Soup
> ¼ cup Land O Lakes no-fat sour cream
> 1¾ cups (one 14½-ounce can) Bavarian-style sauerkraut, drained
> 2 cups (one 16-ounce can) cut green beans, rinsed and drained
> 2 cups hot cooked noodles, rinsed and drained
> ¼ teaspoon black pepper

In a large skillet sprayed with butter-flavored cooking spray,
sauté ham and onion for 5 minutes or until lightly browned. Stir in
mushroom soup and sour cream. Add sauerkraut, green beans,
noodles, and black pepper. Mix well to combine. Lower heat and
simmer for 5 to 6 minutes, stirring occasionally.

HINTS: 1. Regular sauerkraut, ½ teaspoon caraway seeds, and
          1 teaspoon Brown Sugar Twin may be substituted for
          Bavarian sauerkraut.
       2. 1¾ cups uncooked noodles usually cooks to about 2
          cups.

Each serving equals:

HE: 2 Vegetable • 1 Protein • 1 Bread • ½ Slider •
16 Optional Calories

---

244 Calories • 4 gm Fat • 14 gm Protein •
38 gm Carbohydrate • 1,369 mg Sodium •
127 mg Calcium • 5 gm Fiber

DIABETIC: 2 Vegetable • 2 Starch • 1 Meat

Kidney Beans and Ham with Pasta

I've tried to include lots of good-tasting dishes that feature beans in this particular cookbook because fiber is just so important when you're concerned about heart health. Kids like this dish a lot because the shell pasta feels like a trip to the ocean for your taste buds! ☻ Serves 4 (1½ cups)

> 10 ounces (one 16-ounce can) kidney beans, rinsed and drained
> 1 full cup (6 ounces) diced Dubuque 97% fat-free ham or any
>   extra-lean ham
> ½ cup chopped onion
> 1 cup shredded carrots
> 1¾ cups (one 15-ounce can) Hunt's Tomato Sauce
> 2 cups hot cooked macaroni shells, rinsed and drained
> 1 teaspoon dried parsley flakes

In a large skillet sprayed with butter-flavored cooking spray, combine kidney beans, ham, onion, carrots, and tomato sauce. Bring mixture to a boil. Lower heat, cover, and simmer for 20 minutes or until carrots and onion are tender, stirring occasionally. Add macaroni shells and parsley flakes. Mix gently to combine. Continue simmering for 5 minutes or until mixture is heated through, stirring occasionally.

HINT: 1⅓ cups uncooked macaroni usually cooks to about
      2 cups.

Each serving equals:

HE: 2½ Vegetable • 2¼ Protein • 1 Bread

242 Calories • 2 gm Fat • 15 gm Protein •
41 gm Carbohydrate • 1,079 mg Sodium •
37 mg Calcium • 8 gm Fiber

DIABETIC: 2 Vegetable • 2 Starch • 1½ Meat

Cajun Bean Bake

Here's a hearty entree that's full of yummy ingredients and just spicy enough to wake up your mouth with pleasure! Don't be surprised if your family gets up from the table after dining on this dish and starts to dance! This is a meal worth celebrating!

● Serves 6

8 ounces Healthy Choice 97% fat-free frankfurters, diced

1 cup chopped green bell pepper

¼ cup chopped onion

10 ounces (one 16-ounce can) great northern beans, rinsed and drained

1¾ cups (one 14½-ounce can) stewed tomatoes, undrained

2 tablespoons Brown Sugar Twin

1 teaspoon Cajun seasoning

¼ teaspoon black pepper

⅓ cup (1½ ounces) shredded Kraft reduced-fat Cheddar cheese

Preheat oven to 350 degrees. Spray an 8-by-8-inch baking dish with butter-flavored cooking spray. In a large skillet sprayed with butter-flavored cooking spray, sauté frankfurters, green pepper, and onion for 5 minutes or until vegetables are tender. Add great northern beans, undrained stewed tomatoes, Brown Sugar Twin, Cajun seasoning, and black pepper. Mix well to combine. Pour mixture into prepared baking dish. Bake for 30 minutes. Sprinkle Cheddar cheese over top and continue baking for 5 to 6 minutes or until cheese melts. Place baking dish on a wire rack and let set for 5 minutes. Divide into 6 servings.

Each serving equals:

HE: 2 Protein • 1 Vegetable • 5 Optional Calories

138 Calories • 2 gm Fat • 11 gm Protein •
19 gm Carbohydrate • 652 mg Sodium •
116 mg Calcium • 3 gm Fiber

DIABETIC: 1 Meat • 1 Starch • ½ Vegetable

Germantown Shepherd's Pie

Don't mashed potatoes on top make just about anything better? Okay, maybe not pie, but this delightfully tummy-pleasing comfort food works well with just about any kind of meat. In this recipe, I've combined a traditional hot-dog dinner with Cliff's favorite "starch"—and the result is something to sing about.

● Serves 4

> 2 cups (one 16-ounce can) sauerkraut, well drained
> 8 ounces Healthy Choice 97% fat-free frankfurters, diced
> 2 cups (one 16-ounce can) cut green beans, rinsed and drained
> 1/4 teaspoon black pepper
> 1 (10¾-ounce) can Healthy Request Cream of Mushroom Soup ☆
> 1½ cups water
> 1⅓ cups (3 ounces) instant potato flakes
> ⅓ cup Carnation Nonfat Dry Milk Powder
> Dash paprika

Preheat oven to 350 degrees. Spray an 8-by-8-inch baking dish with butter-flavored cooking spray. In a large bowl, combine sauerkraut, frankfurters, green beans, black pepper, and half of mushroom soup. Pour mixture into prepared baking dish. In a medium saucepan, bring water to a boil. Remove from heat. Stir in potato flakes and dry milk powder. Add remaining soup. Mix well to combine. Spread potato mixture evenly over sauerkraut mixture. Lightly sprinkle paprika over top. Bake for 30 to 35 minutes. Place baking dish on a wire rack and let set for 5 minutes. Divide into 4 servings.

Each serving equals:

HE: 2 Vegetable • 1⅓ Protein • 1 Bread •
1/4 Skim Milk • ½ Slider • 1 Optional Calorie

---

215 Calories • 3 gm Fat • 13 gm Protein •
34 gm Carbohydrate • 1,402 mg Sodium •
176 mg Calcium • 5 gm Fiber

DIABETIC: 2 Vegetable • 1½ Meat • 1½ Starch

Desserts

New England Banana Sundae

This is such an easy way to end a meal, but it tastes remarkably special. Did you ever think you'd be gobbling down a sundae topped with syrup and nuts—and calling it healthy? You CAN!

☻ Serves 4

> 2 cups Wells' Blue Bunny sugar- and fat-free vanilla ice cream
> 2 cups (2 medium) diced bananas
> ½ cup Cary's Sugar Free Maple Syrup
> 2 tablespoons (½ ounce) chopped pecans
> ¼ cup Cool Whip Lite

For each sundae, place ½ cup ice cream in dessert dish, sprinkle ½ cup bananas over ice cream, drizzle 2 tablespoons maple syrup over bananas, sprinkle 1½ teaspoons pecans over bananas, and top with 1 tablespoon Cool Whip Lite. Serve at once.

HINTS: 1. If you can't find Wells' Blue Bunny, use any sugar- and fat-free ice cream.
　　　　2. To prevent bananas from turning brown, mix with 1 teaspoon lemon juice or sprinkle with Fruit Fresh.

Each serving equals:

HE: 1 Fruit • ½ Fat • 1 Slider • 10 Optional Calories

211 Calories • 3 gm Fat • 5 gm Protein •
41 gm Carbohydrate • 118 mg Sodium •
126 mg Calcium • 2 gm Fiber

DIABETIC: 1½ Starch/Carbohydrate • 1 Fruit • ½ Fat

Oatmeal Chocolate Chip Cookies

It took a lot of careful testing to figure out how to make a truly delicious healthy cookie, but I bet you'll agree these moist cookies don't taste like diet food! This recipe serves eight, so you can choose how many cookies to make from it. I like the idea of eating three medium-size cookies, but if a giant cookie will please you or your kids, feel free to bake 'em up. You may need to adjust baking time, so keep a close eye on the oven. ❂ Serves 8 (3 each)

¼ cup reduced-calorie margarine

¼ cup unsweetened applesauce

⅔ cup Sugar Twin or Sprinkle Sweet

¼ cup skim milk

1 teaspoon vanilla extract

1 egg, beaten, or equivalent in egg substitute

¾ cup all-purpose flour

1 cup (3 ounces) quick oats

½ teaspoon baking soda

¼ cup (1 ounce) mini chocolate chips

¼ cup (1 ounce) chopped walnuts

Preheat oven to 375 degrees. Spray baking sheets with butter-flavored cooking spray. In a large bowl, combine margarine and applesauce. Stir in sugar substitute, skim milk, and vanilla extract. Add egg. Mix well to combine. Stir in flour, oats, and baking soda. Add chocolate chips and walnuts. Mix gently to combine. Drop by teaspoonful onto prepared baking sheets to form 24 cookies. Bake for 10 to 12 minutes. Place baking sheets on wire racks to cool.

HINT: 32 very small, 16 larger, or 8 very large cookies can be made in place of 24 regular-size ones. Just be sure whatever number you choose to bake can be divided by 8.

Each serving equals:

HE: 1 Bread • 1 Fat • ¼ Protein • ¼ Slider •
13 Optional Calories

150 Calories • 6 gm Fat • 4 gm Protein •
20 gm Carbohydrate • 119 mg Sodium •
24 mg Calcium • 2 gm Fiber

DIABETIC: 1 Starch/Carbohydrate • 1 Fat

Peach Melba Custard

I often joke that my Peach Melba desserts will make you want to sing like the opera singer for whom the dessert was originally invented, Miss Nellie Melba. The blend of peaches and raspberries is surely a combo worth celebrating at the top of your lungs, especially when it's joined by the creamy pudding that accompanies all that lovely fruit.   ☻   Serves 4

> 2 cups (one 16-ounce can) sliced peaches, packed in fruit juice, drained, and ½ cup liquid reserved
> 1 (4-serving) package JELL-O sugar-free vanilla cook-and-serve pudding mix
> ⅔ cup Carnation Nonfat Dry Milk Powder
> 1 cup water
> 1 teaspoon vanilla extract
> 2 tablespoons red raspberry spreadable fruit
> ¼ cup Cool Whip Lite

Evenly divide peaches among 4 dessert dishes. In a medium saucepan, combine dry pudding mix and dry milk powder. Add reserved peach liquid and water. Mix well to combine. Cook over medium heat until mixture thickens and starts to boil, stirring constantly. Remove from heat. Stir in vanilla extract. Evenly spoon hot pudding mixture over peaches. Refrigerate for 30 minutes. Spread 1½ teaspoons raspberry spreadable fruit over pudding layer. Top each with 1 tablespoon Cool Whip Lite. Refrigerate for at least 30 minutes.

Each serving equals:

HE: 1½ Fruit • ½ Skim Milk • ¼ Slider •
8 Optional Calories

---

133 Calories • 1 gm Fat • 4 gm Protein •
27 gm Carbohydrate • 392 mg Sodium •
142 mg Calcium • 1 gm Fiber

DIABETIC: 1½ Fruit •
½ Skim Milk *or* 2 Starch/Carbohydrate

Scalloped Pineapple ❄

This old-fashioned dessert is a kind of pineapple bread pudding made especially moist and delightful with the addition of fat-free mayonnaise, the healthy cook's best baking friend! This makes a wonderful dish for a weekend brunch. ◐ Serves 6

2 cups (two 8-ounce cans) crushed pineapple, packed in fruit juice, undrained
½ cup unsweetened orange juice
3 eggs, beaten, or equivalent in egg substitute
6 slices reduced-calorie bread, cubed
½ cup Sugar Twin or Sprinkle Sweet
2 tablespoons Kraft fat-free mayonnaise
2 tablespoons raisins

Preheat oven to 350 degrees. Spray an 8-by-8-inch baking dish with butter-flavored cooking spray. In a large bowl, combine undrained pineapple, orange juice, eggs, bread cubes, sugar substitute, mayonnaise, and raisins. Pour mixture into prepared baking dish. Bake for 35 to 40 minutes. Place baking dish on a wire rack and let set for 5 minutes. Divide into 6 servings.

Each serving equals:

HE: 1 Fruit • 1 Bread • ½ Protein (limited) • 3 Optional Calories

159 Calories • 3 gm Fat • 6 gm Protein • 27 gm Carbohydrate • 191 mg Sodium • 45 mg Calcium • 3 gm Fiber

DIABETIC: 1 Fruit • 1 Starch • ½ Meat or 2 Starch/Carbohydrate • ½ Meat

Caramel Apricot Rice Pudding ❄

Here's a cozy way to warm hearts on the chilliest winter afternoon: Mix up a soothing rice pudding that's filled with bits of tasty apricot! My daughter, Becky, loves this dish because butterscotch pudding has always been one of her true favorites.

◐ Serves 6

3½ cups water ☆
1 cup (4½ ounces) diced dried apricots
1⅓ cups (4 ounces) uncooked Minute Rice
1 (4-serving) package JELL-O sugar-free instant butterscotch
*   pudding mix*
⅔ cup Carnation Nonfat Dry Milk Powder
¼ cup Cool Whip Free
1 teaspoon vanilla extract

In a medium saucepan, combine 2 cups water and apricots. Bring mixture to a boil. Remove from heat. Stir in uncooked rice. Cover and let set for 15 minutes to cool. In a large bowl, combine dry pudding mix, dry milk powder, and remaining 1½ cups water. Mix well using a wire whisk. Blend in Cool Whip Free and vanilla extract. Fold in cooled rice mixture. Mix gently to combine. Evenly spoon mixture into 6 dessert dishes. Refrigerate for at least 30 minutes.

Each serving equals:

HE: 1 Fruit • ⅔ Bread • ⅓ Skim Milk • ¼ Slider • 2 Optional Calories

100 Calories • 0 gm Fat • 3 gm Protein • 22 gm Carbohydrate • 272 mg Sodium • 100 mg Calcium • 1 gm Fiber

DIABETIC: 1 Fruit • ½ Starch/Carbohydrate

Banana Plantation Rice Pudding

Rice pudding is beloved comfort food in just about every family, but I'm always looking for ways to make what is already luscious even better. This banana dessert is sweet, crunchy, and oh-so-creamy, you'll win fans of all ages! ☻ Serves 6

1 (4-serving) package JELL-O sugar-free instant banana cream
pudding mix
⅔ cup Carnation Nonfat Dry Milk Powder
1½ cups water
¾ cup Cool Whip Free ☆
2 cups (2 medium) diced bananas
3 tablespoons (¾ ounce) chopped pecans
1½ cups cold cooked rice

In a large bowl, combine dry pudding mix, dry milk powder, and water. Mix well using a wire whisk. Blend in ¼ cup Cool Whip Free. Add bananas, pecans, and rice. Mix gently to combine. Evenly spoon mixture into 6 dessert dishes. Top each with 1 tablespoon Cool Whip Free. Refrigerate for at least 1 hour.

HINTS: 1. To prevent bananas from turning brown, mix with 1 teaspoon lemon juice or sprinkle with Fruit Fresh.
2. 1 cup uncooked rice usually cooks to about 1½ cups.

Each serving equals:

HE: ⅔ Fruit • ½ Fat • ½ Bread • ⅓ Skim Milk • ¼ Slider • 12 Optional Calories

175 Calories • 3 gm Fat • 4 gm Protein • 33 gm Carbohydrate • 274 mg Sodium • 100 mg Calcium • 1 gm Fiber

DIABETIC: 1 Fruit • 1 Starch • ½ Fat *or* 2 Starch/Carbohydrate • ½ Fat

Sam's Baked Rice Pudding

Rice pudding is a favorite at the Lund residence, but this baked version is something extra-special. The flavors really mingle in the heat of the oven, making this wonderfully sweet and fragrant. Make sure you put enough water in the baking dish to keep the custard cups from burning on the bottom. (In French, they call this baking "bath" a *bain-marie*.) ☻ Serves 4

1 (4-serving) package JELL-O sugar-free vanilla cook-and-serve pudding mix
⅔ cup Carnation Nonfat Dry Milk Powder

1¾ cups water
1 teaspoon vanilla extract
½ teaspoon apple pie spice
2 cups hot cooked rice
½ cup raisins

Preheat oven to 350 degrees. In a large bowl, combine dry pudding mix, dry milk powder, and water. Mix well using a wire whisk. Blend in vanilla extract and apple pie spice. Add rice and raisins. Mix well to combine. Evenly spoon mixture into four (1-cup) custard dishes. Place custard dishes in an 8-by-8-inch baking dish filled with 1 inch hot water. Bake for 25 to 30 minutes. Place baking dish on a wire rack and let set for 5 minutes. Good served warm or cold.

HINT: 1⅓ cups uncooked rice usually cooks to about 2 cups.

Each serving equals:

HE: 1 Bread • 1 Fruit • ½ Skim Milk • ¼ Slider

196 Calories • 0 gm Fat • 6 gm Protein • 43 gm Carbohydrate • 181 mg Sodium • 153 mg Calcium • 1 gm Fiber

DIABETIC: 1½ Starch • 1 Fruit • ½ Skim Milk *or* 2 Starch/Carbohydrate • 1 Fruit

Sour Cream Raisin Tarts ❄

These individual dessert crusts are great for making treats for a crowd or just for your family. Keep them in your cupboard for culinary emergencies—or if you just got some good news and want to celebrate with a special creamy treat.　　●　　Serves 6

> 1 (4-serving) package JELL-O sugar-free instant vanilla pudding
>   mix
> ⅔ cup Carnation Nonfat Dry Milk Powder
> 1 cup water
> ½ cup Land O Lakes no-fat sour cream
> 1 teaspoon vanilla extract
> ½ cup raisins
> 1 (6 single-serve) package Keebler graham cracker crusts
> 6 tablespoons Cool Whip Lite
> Dash nutmeg

In a large bowl, combine dry pudding mix, dry milk powder, and water. Mix well using a wire whisk. Blend in sour cream and vanilla extract. Add raisins. Mix well to combine. Evenly spoon mixture into graham cracker crusts. Top each with 1 tablespoon Cool Whip Lite and lightly sprinkle with nutmeg.

HINT:　To plump up raisins without "cooking," place in a glass measuring cup and microwave on HIGH for 30 seconds.

Each serving equals:

HE: ⅔ Fruit • ½ Bread • ⅓ Skim Milk • ¼ Slider • 7 Optional Calories

222 Calories • 6 gm Fat • 5 gm Protein • 37 gm Carbohydrate • 439 mg Sodium • 119 mg Calcium • 1 gm Fiber

DIABETIC: 1½ Starch/Carbohydrate • 1 Fruit • 1 Fat

Shortcakes with Strawberry-Rhubarb Banana Sauce

Most restaurant desserts are so high in fat and sugar, I usually pass them up. But I love strawberry shortcake so much I will make an exception for this special treat, only when the berries are really ripe and the shortcake freshly baked. If you want to experience this special pleasure at home, here's a scrumptious way to prepare my favorite treat. ☻ Serves 4

¾ cup Bisquick Reduced Fat Baking Mix

⅓ cup Carnation Nonfat Dry Milk Powder

2 tablespoons Sugar Twin or Sprinkle Sweet

2 tablespoons Kraft fat-free mayonnaise

⅔ cup water ☆

2 cups chopped fresh rhubarb

1 (4-serving) package JELL-O sugar-free strawberry gelatin

1 cup (1 medium) diced banana

1 cup sliced fresh strawberries

¼ cup Cool Whip Lite

Preheat oven to 415 degrees. Spray a baking sheet with butter-flavored cooking spray. In a medium bowl, combine baking mix, dry milk powder, and sugar substitute. Add mayonnaise and ⅓ cup water. Mix well to combine. Drop by spoonfuls onto prepared baking sheet to form 4 shortcakes. Bake for 8 to 12 minutes or until golden brown. Place baking sheet on a wire rack and allow to cool. Meanwhile, in a medium saucepan, combine rhubarb and remaining ⅓ cup water. Cook over medium heat for 6 to 8 minutes or until rhubarb becomes soft, stirring often. Remove from heat. Stir in dry gelatin. Mix well to dissolve gelatin. Add bananas and strawberries. Mix gently to combine. Refrigerate until cooled. For each serving, place 1 shortcake in a dessert dish, spoon about ½ cup rhubarb sauce over top, and garnish with 1 tablespoon Cool Whip Lite.

Each serving equals:

HE: 1 Bread • ¾ Fruit • ½ Vegetable •
¼ Skim Milk • ¼ Slider • 4 Optional Calories

186 Calories • 2 gm Fat • 6 gm Protein •
36 gm Carbohydrate • 415 mg Sodium •
147 mg Calcium • 3 gm Fiber

DIABETIC: 1½ Starch/Carbohydrate • 1 Fruit

Winter Strawberry-Rhubarb Cobbler

We Iowans believe in celebrating the glory of rhubarb all year long, not just in the spring when those lovely stalks are featured at farm stands and markets everywhere. This rich and fruity dessert makes magic with not one but two frozen fruits, so even if you live in Alaska, you can enjoy this tasty dessert in December!

☻ Serves 6

> 1 (4-serving) package JELL-O sugar-free vanilla cook-and-serve
>   pudding mix
> ½ cup water
> ¼ cup Sugar Twin or Sprinkle Sweet ☆
> 3 cups frozen unsweetened strawberries, thawed, coarsely
>   chopped, and undrained
> 3 cups frozen rhubarb, thawed
> 1 (7.5-ounce can) Pillsbury refrigerated buttermilk biscuits
> 1 teaspoon ground cinnamon

Preheat oven to 400 degrees. Spray an 8-by-8-inch baking dish with butter-flavored cooking spray. In a medium saucepan, combine dry pudding mix, water, 3 tablespoons sugar substitute, undrained strawberries, and rhubarb. Cook over medium heat until mixture thickens and starts to boil, stirring constantly. Pour mixture into prepared baking dish. Separate biscuits and cut each into 3 pieces. Evenly sprinkle biscuit pieces over top of rhubarb mixture. In a small bowl, combine remaining 1 tablespoon Sugar Twin and cinnamon. Evenly sprinkle mixture over top of biscuit pieces. Bake for 15 to 20 minutes or until biscuits are golden brown. Place baking dish on a wire rack and let set for 5 minutes. Divide into 6 servings. Good served warm or cold.

Each serving equals:

HE: 1¼ Bread • 1 Vegetable • ½ Fruit •
17 Optional Calories

146 Calories • 2 gm Fat • 3 gm Protein •
29 gm Carbohydrate • 402 mg Sodium •
67 mg Calcium • 5 gm Fiber

DIABETIC: 1 Starch • 1 Fruit *or* 2 Starch/Carbohydrate

Peach Patchwork Cobbler

Is there a man alive who wouldn't trade a kiss for a piece of fresh peach cobbler? If there is, I haven't met him yet! This version makes all those juicy peaches even yummier with a delectable "quilted" topping of golden biscuit bits. Hmm . . . but will two kisses get him seconds? ☻ Serves 6

> 1 (4-serving) package JELL-O sugar-free vanilla cook-and-serve pudding mix
> 1 (4-serving) package JELL-O sugar-free lemon gelatin
> 1¼ cups water
> 3 cups (6 medium) peeled and sliced fresh peaches
> 1 (7.5-ounce) can Pillsbury refrigerated buttermilk biscuits
> ½ teaspoon ground nutmeg
> 2 tablespoons Sugar Twin or Sprinkle Sweet

Preheat oven to 350 degrees. Spray an 8-by-8-inch baking dish with butter-flavored cooking spray. In a large skillet, combine dry pudding mix, dry gelatin, and water. Cook over medium heat until mixture thickens and starts to boil, stirring constantly. Remove from heat. Stir in peaches. Place skillet on a wire rack and allow to cool slightly. Meanwhile, separate biscuits and cut each into 4 pieces. Gently fold biscuit pieces into warm peach mixture. Pour mixture into prepared baking dish. In a small bowl, combine nutmeg and sugar substitute. Evenly sprinkle nutmeg mixture over top. Bake for 45 minutes. Place baking dish on a wire rack and allow to cool. Divide into 6 servings.

HINT: Good cold with 1 tablespoon Cool Whip Lite, or warm with ¼ cup Wells' Blue Bunny sugar- and fat-free vanilla ice cream. If using either, count optional calories accordingly.

Each serving equals:

HE: 1¼ Bread • 1 Fruit • ¼ Slider •
2 Optional Calories

145 Calories • 1 gm Fat • 4 gm Protein •
30 gm Carbohydrate • 417 mg Sodium •
5 mg Calcium • 3 gm Fiber

DIABETIC: 1 Starch • 1 Fruit *or* 2 Starch/Carbohydrate

Apple Valley Cream Pie

Layering flavors is one of my healthy cooking secrets, and you can see how it works in this delectable dessert. Instead of water or milk in the pudding, I use apple juice, stir in some apple pie spice, and of course mix in all those tasty chunks of apple. Make sure you allow enough time for the pie to cool completely before making the topping. ☻ Serves 8

> 1 (4-serving) package JELL-O sugar-free vanilla cook-and-serve
>   pudding mix
> 2 cups unsweetened apple juice ☆
> 1 teaspoon apple pie spice
> 2 cups (4 small) cored, unpeeled, and chopped cooking apples
> 1 teaspoon vanilla extract
> 1 (4-serving) package JELL-O sugar-free instant vanilla pudding
>   mix
> ⅔ cup Carnation Nonfat Dry Milk Powder
> 1 (6-ounce) Keebler graham cracker piecrust
> ¾ cup Cool Whip Lite
> 2 tablespoons (½ ounce) chopped pecans

In a medium saucepan, combine dry cook-and-serve pudding mix and 1 cup apple juice. Add apple pie spice and apples. Cook over medium heat until mixture thickens and apples soften, stirring often. Remove from heat. Stir in vanilla extract. Place saucepan on a wire rack and allow to cool completely. In a medium bowl, combine dry instant pudding mix and dry milk powder. Add remaining 1 cup apple juice. Mix well using a wire whisk. Blend in cooled apple mixture. Spread mixture evenly into piecrust. Refrigerate for at least 2 hours. Spread Cool Whip Lite evenly over set filling. Sprinkle pecans evenly over the top. Refrigerate for at least 15 minutes. Cut into 8 servings.

Each serving equals:

HE: 1 Fruit • ½ Bread • ¼ Fat • ¼ Skim Milk •
1 Slider • 4 Optional Calories

219 Calories • 7 gm Fat • 3 gm Protein •
36 gm Carbohydrate • 390 mg Sodium •
76 mg Calcium • 1 gm Fiber

DIABETIC: 1½ Starch/Carbohydrate • 1 Fruit • 1 Fat

St. Paddy's Chocolate Mint Tarts ❄

Everyone who tries these lovely desserts will surely be convinced they've found the leprechaun's secret stash of gold at the end of the rainbow! They're truly tasty and as colorful as smiling Irish eyes.

◐ Serves 6

> 1 (8-ounce) package Philadelphia fat-free cream cheese
> 1 (4-serving) package JELL-O sugar-free instant chocolate fudge
>   pudding mix
> ⅔ cup Carnation Nonfat Dry Milk Powder
> 1 cup water
> ¾ cup Cool Whip Free ☆
> ¾ teaspoon mint extract ☆
> 1 (6 single-serve) package Keebler graham cracker crusts
> 3 to 4 drops green food coloring
> 1 tablespoon (¼ ounce) mini chocolate chips

In a medium bowl, stir cream cheese with a spoon until soft. Add dry pudding mix, dry milk powder, and water. Mix well using a wire whisk. Blend in ¼ cup Cool Whip Free and ½ teaspoon mint extract. Evenly spoon mixture into graham cracker crusts. In a small bowl, combine remaining ½ cup Cool Whip Free, remaining ¼ teaspoon mint extract, and green food coloring. Spoon scant 1 tablespoon mixture over each tart. Sprinkle ½ teaspoon chocolate chips evenly over each. Refrigerate for at least 30 minutes.

Each serving equals:

HE: ⅔ Protein • ½ Bread • ⅓ Skim Milk • 1 Slider • 16 Optional Calories

---

214 Calories • 6 gm Fat • 10 gm Protein • 30 gm Carbohydrate • 643 mg Sodium • 93 mg Calcium • 1 gm Fiber

---

DIABETIC: 2 Starch/Carbohydrate • 1 Fat

Riviera Strawberry Pie

They're rosy red, they sparkle like gems, and they taste like a piece of heaven—I MUST be talking about strawberries, my best of all fruits! This luscious pie takes what's already fabulous and makes it so good you'll be smiling all day long. And can you believe that a serving of this tasty dessert is less than 200 calories? It's true!

☻ Serves 8

4 cups sliced fresh strawberries ☆
1 (6-ounce) Keebler shortbread piecrust
¾ cup water
1 (4-serving) package JELL-O sugar-free vanilla cook-and-serve
*   pudding mix*
1 (4-serving) package JELL-O sugar-free strawberry gelatin
1 (8-ounce) package Philadelphia fat-free cream cheese
½ teaspoon almond extract
½ cup Cool Whip Lite

Layer half of strawberries in bottom of piecrust. Mash remaining strawberries with a potato masher or fork. In a medium saucepan, combine mashed strawberries, water, dry pudding mix, and dry gelatin. Cook over medium heat until mixture thickens and starts to boil, stirring constantly. Remove from heat. Add cream cheese and almond extract. Mix well with a wire whisk until well blended. Pour hot mixture evenly over strawberries in piecrust. Refrigerate for at least 2 hours. Cut into 8 servings. When serving, top each piece with 1 tablespoon Cool Whip Lite.

Each serving equals:

HE: ½ Bread • ½ Fruit • ½ Protein • ¾ Slider • 11 Optional Calories

---

169 Calories • 5 gm Fat • 6 gm Protein •
25 gm Carbohydrate • 350 mg Sodium •
10 mg Calcium • 2 gm Fiber

DIABETIC: 1 Starch • 1 Fat • ½ Fruit •
½ Meat *or* 1½ Starch/Carbohydrate • 1 Fat • ½ Meat

Fresh Peach-Blueberry Pie

What a great Fourth of July or end-of-summer party dessert this delectable pie will make! Pick your ripest peaches and the sweetest blueberries you can find, then tumble them together into a waiting piecrust and top with a sweet and creamy topping. This put a real smile on the fruit-stained faces of my grandbabies, Zach and Josh!

☺ Serves 8

> 2 cups (4 medium) peeled and sliced fresh peaches
> 1 (6-ounce) Keebler graham cracker piecrust
> 1½ cups fresh blueberries
> 1 (4-serving) package JELL-O sugar-free lemon gelatin
> 1 (4-serving) package JELL-O sugar-free vanilla cook-and-serve pudding mix
> 1½ cups water
> ¼ teaspoon ground nutmeg
> ½ cup Cool Whip Lite

Layer peaches in bottom of piecrust. Evenly sprinkle blueberries over peaches. In a medium saucepan, combine dry gelatin, dry pudding mix, and water. Cook over medium heat until mixture thickens and starts to boil, stirring constantly. Remove from heat. Stir in nutmeg. Spoon hot mixture evenly over fruit. Refrigerate for at least 2 hours. Cut into 8 servings. When serving, top each piece with 1 tablespoon Cool Whip Lite.

Each serving equals:

HE: ¾ Fruit • ½ Bread • ¾ Slider • 15 Optional Calories

173 Calories • 5 gm Fat • 2 gm Protein • 30 gm Carbohydrate • 291 mg Sodium • 5 mg Calcium • 2 gm Fiber

DIABETIC: 1 Fruit • 1 Starch • 1 Fat

Angel Delight Pie

Even if you've never made a pie before, you'll convince your family you've been touched by an angel when you serve this scrumptious coconutty treat! It looks and tastes like a bit of heaven. It tastes as if it's *loaded* with high-fat goodies like pecans, but it's not—so you can enjoy this without a bit of guilt. ❂ Serves 8

1 (4-serving) package JELL-O sugar-free vanilla cook-and-serve pudding mix
⅔ cup Carnation Nonfat Dry Milk Powder
1¼ cups water
1 teaspoon coconut extract
1 (8-ounce) package Philadelphia fat-free cream cheese
1 cup raisins
2 tablespoons (½ ounce) chopped pecans
2 tablespoons flaked coconut
1 (6-ounce) Keebler shortbread piecrust

In a medium saucepan, combine dry pudding mix, dry milk powder, and water. Cook over medium heat until mixture thickens and starts to boil, stirring constantly. Remove from heat. Add coconut extract and cream cheese. Blend well using a wire whisk. Gently fold in raisins, pecans, and coconut. Spread mixture evenly into piecrust. Refrigerate for at least 2 hours. Cut into 8 servings.

HINT: To plump up raisins without "cooking," place in a glass measuring cup and microwave on HIGH for 45 seconds.

Each serving equals:

HE: 1 Fruit • ½ Bread • ½ Protein • ¼ Skim Milk • ¼ Fat • ¾ Slider • 4 Optional Calories

---

226 Calories • 6 gm Fat • 7 gm Protein • 36 gm Carbohydrate • 358 mg Sodium • 79 mg Calcium • 1 gm Fiber

---

DIABETIC: 1½ Starch/Carbohydrate • 1 Fruit • 1 Fat • ½ Meat

Mocha-Banana Cream Pie

Mocha is the favorite flavor of many of our Healthy Exchanges staffers, so I created this pie for one of our many birthday celebrations at the "House That Recipes Built." This creamy dish is jam-packed with so many good things—nuts, chips, bananas—that every bite will make you cheer. It's a true showstopper!

☺ Serves 8

> 2 cups (2 medium) sliced bananas
> 1 (6-ounce) Keebler chocolate piecrust
> 1 (4-serving) package JELL-O sugar-free instant chocolate fudge
>   pudding mix
> 1 cup Carnation Nonfat Dry Milk Powder ☆
> 1 teaspoon instant coffee crystals
> ¾ cup Yoplait plain fat-free yogurt
> 1¾ cups water ☆
> 1 teaspoon almond extract
> 1 (4-serving) package JELL-O sugar-free instant banana cream
>   pudding mix
> 1 tablespoon (¼ ounce) chopped almonds
> 1 tablespoon (¼ ounce) mini chocolate chips

Layer bananas in bottom of piecrust. In a medium bowl, combine dry chocolate fudge pudding mix, ⅓ cup dry milk powder, and coffee crystals. Add yogurt and ¾ cup water. Mix well using a wire whisk. Blend in almond extract. Spread mixture evenly over bananas. Refrigerate while preparing banana cream mixture. In another medium bowl, combine dry banana cream pudding mix, remaining ⅔ cup dry milk powder, and remaining 1 cup water. Mix well using a wire whisk. Spread banana cream mixture evenly over chocolate layer. Sprinkle almonds and chocolate chips evenly over top. Refrigerate for at least 30 minutes. Cut into 8 servings.

HINT: To prevent bananas from turning brown, mix with 1 teaspoon lemon juice or sprinkle with Fruit Fresh.

Each serving equals:

HE: ½ Bread • ½ Skim Milk • ¼ Fruit • 1 Slider • 9 Optional Calories

226 Calories • 6 gm Fat • 6 gm Protein • 37 gm Carbohydrate • 498 mg Sodium • 152 mg Calcium • 1 gm Fiber

DIABETIC: 1 Starch • 1 Fat • ½ Skim Milk • ½ Fruit *or* 2 Starch/Carbohydrate • 1 Fat

The Governor's Banana Cream Pie

When I was appointed to Iowa's Rural Health and Primary Care Committee by Governor Branstad of Iowa, I responded as I often do on special occasions—I created a pie! Since the governor's favorite flavor is banana (yes, I called and checked with his staff), I knew this pie would easily win his vote!   ☻   Serves 8

> 2 cups (2 medium) sliced bananas
> 1 (6-ounce) Keebler graham cracker piecrust
> 1 (4-serving) package JELL-O sugar-free instant vanilla pudding
>   mix
> 1⅓ cups Carnation Nonfat Dry Milk Powder ☆
> 2⅓ cups water ☆
> 1 teaspoon vanilla extract
> 1 (4-serving) package JELL-O sugar-free instant banana cream
>   pudding mix
> ½ cup Cool Whip Free
> 1 tablespoon purchased graham cracker crumbs or one (2½-inch)
>   graham cracker square made into crumbs

Layer bananas in bottom of piecrust. In a medium bowl, combine dry vanilla pudding mix, ⅔ cup dry milk powder, and 1⅓ cups water. Mix well using a wire whisk. Blend in vanilla extract. Pour mixture evenly over bananas. Refrigerate while preparing topping. In a medium bowl, combine dry banana cream pudding mix, remaining ⅔ cup dry milk powder, and remaining 1 cup water. Mix well using a wire whisk. Blend in Cool Whip Free. Spread mixture evenly over set vanilla layer. Sprinkle graham cracker crumbs evenly over top. Refrigerate for at least 30 minutes. Cut into 8 servings.

HINT: To prevent bananas from turning brown, mix with 1 teaspoon lemon juice or sprinkle with Fruit Fresh.

Each serving equals:

HE: ½ Bread • ½ Fruit • ½ Skim Milk • 1 Slider • 6 Optional Calories

217 Calories • 5 gm Fat • 5 gm Protein • 38 gm Carbohydrate • 541 mg Sodium • 141 mg Calcium • 1 gm Fiber

DIABETIC: 1½ Starch • ½ Fruit • ½ Skim Milk • ½ Fat *or* 2 Starch/Carbohydrate • ½ Skim Milk • ½ Fat

Mandarin Orange–Pineapple Pie

This pie is really lovely to look at, but it's the blend of fruit flavors that makes it truly special. My grandsons, Zach and Josh, are super fans of pineapple and mandarin oranges, so when I asked them to help me test this pie, they smiled from ear to ear. Then they gobbled it down and gave me an even bigger smile. I guess they liked it! ☻ Serves 8

1 (4-serving) package JELL-O sugar-free orange gelatin
1 (4-serving) package JELL-O sugar-free vanilla cook-and-serve pudding mix
⅔ cup Carnation Nonfat Dry Milk Powder
1 cup unsweetened orange juice
1 cup (one 8-ounce can) crushed pineapple, packed in fruit juice, undrained
1½ teaspoons coconut extract ☆
1 cup (one 11-ounce can) mandarin oranges, rinsed and drained
1 (6-ounce) Keebler graham cracker piecrust
¾ cup Cool Whip Free
2 tablespoons flaked coconut

In a medium saucepan, combine dry gelatin, dry pudding mix, and dry milk powder. Add orange juice and undrained pineapple. Mix well to combine. Cook over medium heat until mixture thickens and starts to boil, stirring constantly. Remove from heat. Stir in ½ teaspoon coconut extract and mandarin oranges. Place saucepan on a wire rack and allow to cool for 5 minutes. Spread partially cooled mixture into piecrust. Refrigerate for 2 hours or until filling is firm. In a small bowl, combine Cool Whip Free and remaining 1 teaspoon coconut extract. Spread topping mixture evenly over pie filling. Sprinkle coconut evenly over top. Refrigerate for at least 30 minutes. Cut into 8 servings.

Each serving equals:

HE: ¾ Fruit • ½ Bread • ¼ Skim Milk • 1 Slider

201 Calories • 5 gm Fat • 4 gm Protein •
35 gm Carbohydrate • 367 mg Sodium •
79 mg Calcium • 1 gm Fiber

DIABETIC: 1 Fruit • 1 Starch •
1 Fat *or* 2 Starch/Carbohydrate

Chocolate-Covered Cherry Cordial Pie

Mmm . . . just close your eyes and think of how a chocolate-covered cherry tastes when you bite into it. Now hold that thought—and stir up this luscious pie! Besides being truly beautiful to look at, this dessert tastes oh-so-yummy! It's perfect for a party or any time you want to tell someone you love how much you care.

🗨 Serves 8

> 12 maraschino cherries ☆
> 1 (8-ounce) package Philadelphia fat-free cream cheese
> ¾ cup Cool Whip Free ☆
> Sugar substitute to equal 2 tablespoons sugar
> 2 or 3 drops red food coloring
> 1 (6-ounce) Keebler chocolate piecrust
> 1 (4-serving) package JELL-O sugar-free instant chocolate fudge
>   pudding mix
> ⅔ cup Carnation Nonfat Dry Milk Powder
> 1¼ cups water
> 1 teaspoon brandy extract

Set aside 4 maraschino cherries. Coarsely chop remaining 8 maraschino cherries. In a medium bowl, stir cream cheese with a spoon until soft. Stir in ¼ cup Cool Whip Free and sugar substitute. Add chopped maraschino cherries and red food coloring. Mix gently to combine. Spread mixture evenly into piecrust. In a large bowl, combine dry pudding mix, dry milk powder, and water. Mix well using a wire whisk. Blend in brandy extract. Pour chocolate mixture evenly over cream cheese mixture. Refrigerate for 10 minutes. Evenly drop remaining ½ cup Cool Whip Free by spoonfuls to form 8 mounds. Cut remaining 4 maraschino cherries in half. Garnish each mound with a cherry half. Refrigerate for at least 1 hour. Cut into 8 servings.

Each serving equals:

HE: ½ Bread • ½ Protein • ¼ Skim Milk • 1 Slider •
15 Optional Calories

---

194 Calories • 6 gm Fat • 7 gm Protein •
28 gm Carbohydrate • 469 mg Sodium •
69 mg Calcium • 0 gm Fiber

DIABETIC: 2 Starch • ½ Meat • ½ Fat

Chocolate Pecan Layered Pie

Chocolate, chocolate, and more chocolate—if that's not a recipe for dessert delight, I don't know what is! Add some pecans and whipped topping, and you've got a fabulous treat fit for an anniversary or birthday celebration. ☻ Serves 8

> 1 (4-serving) package JELL-O sugar-free chocolate cook-and-serve pudding mix
>
> 1⅓ cups Carnation Nonfat Dry Milk Powder ☆
>
> 2¼ cups water ☆
>
> ¼ cup (1 ounce) chopped pecans
>
> 1 teaspoon vanilla extract
>
> 1 (6-ounce) Keebler chocolate piecrust
>
> 1 (4-serving) package JELL-O sugar-free instant chocolate pudding mix
>
> 1 cup Cool Whip Free ☆
>
> 1 tablespoon (¼ ounce) mini chocolate chips

In a medium saucepan, combine dry cook-and-serve pudding mix, ⅔ cup dry milk powder, and 1 cup water. Cook over medium heat until mixture thickens and just starts to boil, stirring constantly. Remove from heat. Stir in pecans and vanilla extract. Place saucepan on a wire rack and allow to cool for 5 minutes. Spread partially cooled mixture evenly into piecrust. Cover and refrigerate for at least 30 minutes. In a medium bowl, combine dry instant pudding mix, remaining ⅔ cup dry milk powder, and remaining 1¼ cups water. Mix well using a wire whisk. Blend in ½ cup Cool Whip Free. Spread mixture evenly over set pecan layer. Refrigerate for 10 minutes. Spread remaining ½ cup Cool Whip Free evenly over set chocolate layer. Sprinkle chocolate chips evenly over top. Refrigerate for at least 1 hour. Cut into 8 servings.

Each serving equals:

HE: ½ Bread • ½ Skim Milk • ½ Fat • 1 Slider • 17 Optional Calories

204 Calories • 8 gm Fat • 5 gm Protein • 28 gm Carbohydrate • 225 mg Sodium • 141 mg Calcium • 1 gm Fiber

DIABETIC: 2 Starch/Carbohydrate • 1 Fat

Crossroads Pie

I created this pie in honor of the groundbreaking ceremony for the "House That Recipes Built," which was built in DeWitt's Industrial Park on land we bought from Crossroads Development. This festive pie is just chock-full of fruit, chock-full of flavor, and definitely a treat in every sense of the word! This is one recipe I truly enjoyed testing—maybe because of the aroma in my kitchen while I was cooking the cherries . . . wow! ☻ Serves 8

1 (4-serving) package JELL-O sugar-free cherry gelatin

1 (4-serving) package JELL-O sugar-free vanilla cook-and-serve pudding mix

2 cups (one 16-ounce can) tart red cherries, packed in water, drained, and ½ cup liquid reserved

1¾ cups water ☆

1½ teaspoons coconut extract ☆

1 (6-ounce) Keebler graham cracker piecrust

1 (4-serving) package JELL-O sugar-free instant vanilla pudding mix

⅔ cup Carnation Nonfat Dry Milk Powder

¾ cup Cool Whip Free

1 cup (one 8-ounce can) crushed pineapple, packed in fruit juice, drained

2 tablespoons flaked coconut

In a medium saucepan, combine dry gelatin and dry cook-and-serve pudding mix. Add cherries, reserved cherry liquid and ½ cup water. Mix well to combine. Cook over medium heat until mixture thickens and starts to boil, stirring often and being careful not to crush the cherries. Remove from heat. Stir in ½ teaspoon coconut extract. Pour hot mixture evenly into piecrust. Refrigerate for at least 1 hour. In a medium bowl, combine dry instant pudding mix, dry milk powder, and remaining 1¼ cups water. Mix well using a wire whisk. Spread pudding mixture evenly over set cherry filling. In a medium bowl, combine Cool Whip Free, drained pineapple, and remaining 1 teaspoon coconut extract. Spread topping mixture evenly over pudding layer. Sprinkle coconut evenly over top. Refrigerate for at least 1 hour. Cut into 8 servings.

Each serving equals:

HE: ¾ Fruit • ½ Bread • ¼ Skim Milk • 1 Slider •
13 Optional Calories

218 Calories • 6 gm Fat • 4 gm Protein •
37 gm Carbohydrate • 534 mg Sodium •
80 mg Calcium • 1 gm Fiber

DIABETIC: 1½ Starch/Carbohydrate • 1 Fruit • 1 Fat

Barbara's Heavenly Chocolate Pie

✳

Here's a perfect example of how a chance remark helped me create a mouth-watering new pie. My friend Barbara told me about an ice cream flavor she loved, a rich chocolate that also included orange bits and chocolate chips. *Voilà!* The pie began appearing in my mind, the chocolate and orange blending deliciously together. Barbara loved the result, and I hope you will, too! ☻ Serves 8

1 (4-serving) package JELL-O sugar-free instant chocolate fudge pudding mix
⅔ cup Carnation Nonfat Dry Milk Powder
1⅓ cups water
1 cup Cool Whip Free ☆
1 cup (one 11-ounce can) mandarin oranges, rinsed and drained

1 (6-ounce) Keebler chocolate piecrust
1 (4-serving) package JELL-O sugar-free orange gelatin
1 teaspoon coconut extract
2 tablespoons flaked coconut
1 tablespoon (¼ ounce) mini chocolate chips

In a large bowl, combine dry pudding mix, dry milk powder, and water. Mix well using a wire whisk. Blend in ¼ cup Cool Whip Free and mandarin oranges. Spread mixture evenly into piecrust. Refrigerate while preparing topping. In a small bowl, combine remaining ¾ cup Cool Whip Free, dry gelatin, and coconut extract. Spread topping mixture evenly over set filling. Sprinkle coconut and chocolate chips evenly over top. Refrigerate for at least 1 hour. Cut into 8 servings.

Each serving equals:

HE: ½ Bread • ¼ Skim Milk • ¼ Fruit • 1 Slider • 16 Optional Calories

182 Calories • 6 gm Fat • 4 gm Protein • 28 gm Carbohydrate • 333 mg Sodium • 73 mg Calcium • 1 gm Fiber

DIABETIC: 2 Starch/Carbohydrate • 1 Fat

Triple Layer Pumpkin-Pecan Pie

It's easy, easy, oh-so-easy, but better still, it's three-three-three delicious layers in one healthy pie! My daughter, Becky, lives far away,
but this would be the perfect dessert to serve the next time she and
her husband, John, come home to DeWitt!   ☻   Serves 8

1 (8-ounce) package Philadelphia fat-free cream cheese
2 tablespoons Sugar Twin or Sprinkle Sweet
1 teaspoon vanilla extract
1 cup Cool Whip Free ☆
¼ cup (1 ounce) chopped pecans ☆
1 (6-ounce) Keebler graham cracker piecrust
1 (4-serving) package JELL-O sugar-free instant butterscotch
    pudding mix
⅔ cup Carnation Nonfat Dry Milk Powder
¾ cup + 2 tablespoons water
2 cups (one 16-ounce can) pumpkin
1½ teaspoons pumpkin pie spice

In a medium bowl, stir cream cheese with a spoon until soft.
Add sugar substitute and vanilla extract. Mix gently to combine.
Stir in ¼ cup Cool Whip Free and 2 tablespoons chopped pecans.
Spread mixture evenly into piecrust. In a large bowl, combine dry
pudding mix and dry milk powder. Add water and pumpkin. Mix
well using a wire whisk. Blend in pumpkin pie spice and ¼ cup
Cool Whip Free. Spread pumpkin mixture evenly over cream
cheese layer. Spread remaining ½ cup Cool Whip Free over pumpkin layer. Sprinkle remaining 2 tablespoons pecans over top. Refrigerate for at least 2 hours. Cut into 8 servings.

Each serving equals:

HE: ½ Bread • ½ Protein • ½ Vegetable • ½ Fat •
¼ Skim Milk • ¾ Slider • 19 Optional Calories

228 Calories • 8 gm Fat • 8 gm Protein •
31 gm Carbohydrate • 514 mg Sodium •
89 mg Calcium • 3 gm Fiber

DIABETIC: 2 Starch • 1 Fat • ½ Meat

Blender Key Lime Pie

Sure, it would be nice if we could all fly off to Key West on a moment's notice to gobble down that island's renowned lime pie. Since we can't, why not take a culinary journey instead by blending up this tart and creamy pie? Can't you just feel that sunshine on your shoulders? ☻ Serves 8

¾ cup boiling water
1 (4-serving) package JELL-O sugar-free lime gelatin
1 tablespoon lime juice
¾ cup cold water
1 (4-serving) package JELL-O sugar-free instant vanilla pudding mix
1⅓ cups Carnation Nonfat Dry Milk Powder
Sugar substitute to equal 2 tablespoons sugar
1 (6-ounce) Keebler graham cracker piecrust
½ cup Cool Whip Lite
Thin lime slices (optional)

In a blender container, combine boiling water, dry gelatin, and lime juice. Cover and process on HIGH for 20 seconds or until mixture is well blended. Add cold water, dry pudding mix, dry milk powder, and sugar substitute. Re-cover and process on BLEND for 30 seconds or until mixture is smooth. Pour mixture evenly into piecrust. Refrigerate for at least 2 hours. Cut into 8 servings. When serving, top each piece with 1 tablespoon Cool Whip Lite and a lime slice.

Each serving equals:

HE: ½ Bread • ½ Skim Milk • ¾ Slider •
17 Optional Calories

174 Calories • 6 gm Fat • 6 gm Protein •
24 gm Carbohydrate • 389 mg Sodium •
139 mg Calcium • 1 gm Fiber

DIABETIC: 1½ Starch/Carbohydrate • 1 Fat
or 1 Starch/Carbohydrate • 1 Fat • ½ Skim Milk

Ruby Rhubarb Cheesecake

Out here in Iowa, rhubarb shows up in the market during May, and for the next few months, we Iowans just can't get enough of this wonderful fruit that always blends beautifully with strawberries. Here's a cheesecake that celebrates this scrumptious and beloved fruit in a dessert that's delightfully rich and oh-so-pretty, too.

◐ Serves 8

2 cups chopped fresh rhubarb
⅓ cup water
1 (4-serving) package JELL-O sugar-free strawberry gelatin
2 (8-ounce) packages Philadelphia fat-free cream cheese
⅔ cup Carnation Nonfat Dry Milk Powder
1 (4-serving) package JELL-O sugar-free instant vanilla pudding mix
¾ cup Cool Whip Free ☆
1 (6-ounce) Keebler shortbread piecrust

In a medium saucepan, combine rhubarb and water. Cover and cook over medium heat for 5 to 8 minutes or until rhubarb becomes soft, stirring often. Remove from heat. Stir in dry gelatin. Mix well to dissolve gelatin. Cool, uncovered, for 10 minutes. In a large bowl, stir cream cheese with a spoon until soft. Add dry milk powder, dry pudding mix, and cooled rhubarb sauce. Mix well using a wire whisk. Blend in ¼ cup Cool Whip Free. Spread mixture evenly into piecrust. Cover and refrigerate for at least 2 hours. Cut into 8 servings. When serving, top each piece with 1 tablespoon Cool Whip Free.

Each serving equals:

HE: 1 Protein • ½ Bread • ½ Vegetable •
¼ Skim Milk • ¾ Slider • 19 Optional Calories

201 Calories • 5 gm Fat • 12 gm Protein •
27 gm Carbohydrate • 703 mg Sodium •
95 mg Calcium • 1 gm Fiber

DIABETIC: 2 Starch/Carbohydrate • 1 Meat

Peanut Butter and Jelly Cheesecake Pie

I figured there had to be a wonderful dessert in America's favorite kids' sandwich—and this is it! My testers are strawberry fans, but this would also be good with grape or even boysenberry, don't you think? ☻ Serves 8

1 (8-ounce) package Philadelphia fat-free cream cheese
¼ cup Peter Pan reduced-fat peanut butter
1 (4-serving) package JELL-O sugar-free instant vanilla pudding mix
⅔ cup Carnation Nonfat Dry Milk Powder
1 cup water
1 cup Cool Whip Free ☆
1 teaspoon vanilla extract
1 (6-ounce) Keebler graham cracker piecrust
½ cup strawberry spreadable fruit

In a medium bowl, stir cream cheese and peanut butter with a spoon until soft. Add dry pudding mix, dry milk powder, and water. Mix well using a wire whisk. Blend in ¼ cup Cool Whip Free and vanilla extract. Spread mixture into piecrust. Refrigerate while preparing topping. In a small bowl, stir spreadable fruit until softened. Stir in remaining ¾ cup Cool Whip Free. Spread mixture evenly over top. Refrigerate for at least 1 hour. Cut into 8 servings.

Each serving equals:

HE: 1½ Protein • 1 Fruit • ½ Fat • ½ Bread • ¼ Skim Milk • ¾ Slider • 18 Optional Calories

260 Calories • 8 gm Fat • 9 gm Protein • 38 gm Carbohydrate • 436 mg Sodium • 69 mg Calcium • 1 gm Fiber

DIABETIC: 1½ Meat • 1 Fruit • 1 Starch • ½ Fat

Partyline Kahlua Cheesecake ❄

When I appeared on a program called *Partyline* in Youngstown, Ohio, I created this special cheesecake—and everyone at the station gave it top ratings! I named it "kahlua" after the famous coffee liqueur, but it gets its rich flavor from non-alcoholic coffee alone.

☯ Serves 8

> 2 (8-ounce) packages Philadelphia fat-free cream cheese
> 1 (4-serving) package JELL-O sugar-free instant vanilla pudding mix
> ⅔ cup Carnation Nonfat Dry Milk Powder
> 1 cup cold coffee
> 1 teaspoon coconut extract
> ¼ cup Cool Whip Free
> 2 tablespoons (½ ounce) chopped pecans
> 2 tablespoons (½ ounce) mini chocolate chips
> 1 (6-ounce) Keebler chocolate piecrust
> 2 tablespoons flaked coconut

In a medium bowl, stir cream cheese with a spoon until soft. Add dry pudding mix, dry milk powder, and cold coffee. Mix well using a wire whisk. Blend in coconut extract and Cool Whip Free. Add pecans and chocolate chips. Mix well to combine. Spread mixture evenly into piecrust. Sprinkle coconut evenly over top. Refrigerate for at least 2 hours. Cut into 8 servings.

Each serving equals:

HE: 1 Protein • ½ Bread • ¼ Skim Milk • ¼ Fat • 1 Slider

---

223 Calories • 7 gm Fat • 12 gm Protein •
28 gm Carbohydrate • 678 mg Sodium •
81 mg Calcium • 1 gm Fiber

DIABETIC: 1½ Starch • 1 Meat • 1 Fat

Chocolate Raspberry Cheesecake

Here's one of the prettiest cheesecakes I've ever created, and it definitely tastes as fantastic as it looks! I could see serving this for a Valentine's Day dinner when romance is on the menu.

● Serves 8

> 2 (8-ounce) packages Philadelphia fat-free cream cheese
> 1 (4-serving) package JELL-O sugar-free instant vanilla pudding mix
> 1⅓ cups Carnation Nonfat Dry Milk Powder ☆
> 2¼ cups water ☆
> 1½ teaspoons coconut extract ☆
> ¼ cup Cool Whip Free
> 1½ cups frozen unsweetened raspberries, thawed and well drained
> 1 (6-ounce) Keebler chocolate piecrust
> 1 (4-serving) package JELL-O sugar-free chocolate cook-and-serve pudding mix
> 2 tablespoons flaked coconut

In a large bowl, stir cream cheese with a spoon until soft. Add dry instant pudding mix, ⅔ cup dry milk powder, and 1 cup water. Mix well using a wire whisk. Blend in ½ teaspoon coconut extract and Cool Whip Free. Gently fold in raspberries. Spread mixture into piecrust. Refrigerate while preparing sauce. In a medium saucepan, combine dry cook-and-serve pudding mix, remaining ⅔ cup dry milk powder, and remaining 1¼ cups water. Cook over medium heat until mixture thickens and starts to boil, stirring constantly. Remove from heat. Stir in remaining 1 teaspoon coconut extract. Cool for 5 minutes, stirring often. Spoon chocolate mixture over top of cheesecake. Refrigerate for at least 1 hour. Sprinkle coconut evenly over top. Cut into 8 servings.

HINT: Fresh raspberries may be substituted for frozen.

Each serving equals:

HE: 1 Protein • ½ Bread • ½ Skim Milk • ¼ Fruit •
1 Slider • 3 Optional Calories

242 Calories • 6 gm Fat • 14 gm Protein •
33 gm Carbohydrate • 736 mg Sodium •
144 mg Calcium • 1 gm Fiber

DIABETIC: 2 Starch • 1 Meat • 1 Fat

Blueberry Cheesecake Dessert

Graham crackers have magic in them, did you know that? Without a bit of shortening, they can easily be transformed into a tasty crust worthy of the yummiest cheesecake! This soul-pleasing dessert can be stirred up all year round because it's made with frozen berries. Mmm-hmm—good! ○ Serves 8

12 (2½-inch) graham cracker squares
2 (8-ounce) packages Philadelphia fat-free cream cheese
Sugar substitute to equal 3 tablespoons sugar
1 teaspoon vanilla extract
1 cup Cool Whip Free
1 (4-serving) package JELL-O sugar-free lemon gelatin
1 (4-serving) package JELL-O sugar-free vanilla cook-and-serve
*   pudding mix*
½ teaspoon apple pie spice
¾ cup water
3 cups frozen blueberries, thawed, and ¼ cup juice reserved
2 tablespoons lemon juice

Preheat oven to 350 degrees. Evenly arrange graham crackers in a 9-by-13-inch cake pan, breaking as necessary to fit. Bake for 4 minutes. Place cake pan on a wire rack and allow to cool. Meanwhile, in a large bowl, stir cream cheese with a spoon until soft. Add sugar substitute, vanilla extract, and Cool Whip Free. Pour over graham crackers and refrigerate while preparing topping. In a medium saucepan, combine dry gelatin, dry pudding mix, and apple pie spice. Add water, reserved blueberry juice, and lemon juice. Cook over medium heat until mixture thickens and starts to boil, stirring constantly. Add blueberries. Mix gently to combine. Continue cooking for about 5 minutes, being careful not to crush blueberries. Place saucepan on a wire rack and allow to cool for 15 minutes. Spread cooled blueberry mixture over cream cheese layer. Refrigerate for at least 2 hours. Cut into 8 servings.

Each serving equals:

HE: 1 Protein • ½ Bread • ½ Fruit • ¼ Slider •
12 Optional Calories

---

129 Calories • 1 gm Fat • 9 gm Protein •
21 gm Carbohydrate • 467 mg Sodium •
4 mg Calcium • 2 gm Fiber

DIABETIC: 1 Meat • 1 Starch/Carbohydrate • ½ Fruit

Newsletter Center Rhubarb Dessert

My newsletter takes a lot of help to get out each month, and so I try to keep spirits high at the newsletter center by serving them some of my tastiest desserts. And because rhubarb is Iowa's unofficial state fruit, I stirred up this dish to celebrate everyone's favorite flavor! ☻ Serves 8

> 12 (2½-inch) graham cracker squares ☆
> 1 (4-serving) package JELL-O sugar-free vanilla cook-and-serve
>   pudding mix
> 2¼ cups water ☆
> 4 cups chopped fresh rhubarb
> 1 (4-serving) package JELL-O sugar-free strawberry gelatin
> ½ cup (1 ounce) miniature marshmallows
> 1 (4-serving) package JELL-O sugar-free instant vanilla pudding
>   mix
> ⅔ cup Carnation Nonfat Dry Milk Powder
> ½ cup Cool Whip Free
> 1 teaspoon vanilla extract

Place 9 graham crackers in a 9-by-9-inch cake pan. In a medium saucepan, combine dry cook-and-serve pudding mix, ¾ cup water, and rhubarb. Cook over medium heat for 10 to 15 minutes or until rhubarb softens, stirring often. Remove from heat. Stir in dry gelatin. Mix well to dissolve gelatin. Place saucepan on a wire rack and allow to cool for 10 minutes. Spoon mixture evenly over crackers. Cover and refrigerate for 1 hour. Sprinkle marshmallows evenly over top. In a medium bowl, combine dry instant pudding mix, dry milk powder, and remaining 1½ cups water. Mix well using a wire whisk. Blend in Cool Whip Free and vanilla extract. Pour mixture evenly over marshmallows. Crush remaining 3 graham crackers and sprinkle crumbs evenly over top of pudding layer. Cover and refrigerate for at least 30 minutes. Cut into 8 servings.

Each serving equals:

HE: 1 Vegetable • ½ Bread • ¼ Skim Milk •
½ Slider • 2 Optional Calories

101 Calories • 1 gm Fat • 3 gm Protein •
20 gm Carbohydrate • 320 mg Sodium •
122 mg Calcium • 1 gm Fiber

DIABETIC: 1½ Starch/Carbohydrate

French Apple Dessert

This recipe will fill your house with a scrumptious aroma as the apple pastry bakes! What a wonderful way to welcome card party guests to your house—just put this into the oven as your friends arrive . . . then wait for the compliments! 🌑 Serves 8

> 3 cups (6 small) cored, unpeeled, and thinly sliced
>   cooking apples
> 2 teaspoons apple pie spice
> ⅔ cup Carnation Nonfat Dry Milk Powder
> ¾ cup water
> 2 eggs or equivalent in egg substitute
> ½ cup Sugar Twin or Sprinkle Sweet
> 1½ cups Bisquick Reduced Fat Baking Mix ☆
> ¼ cup (1 ounce) chopped pecans
> ¼ cup Brown Sugar Twin
> 1 tablespoon + 1 teaspoon reduced-calorie margarine

Preheat oven to 350 degrees. Spray a 9-by-9-inch cake pan with butter-flavored cooking spray. Evenly arrange apples in cake pan. In a blender container, combine apple pie spice, dry milk powder, water, eggs, sugar substitute, and ¾ cup baking mix. Cover and process on HIGH for 15 to 20 seconds or until smooth. Pour mixture over apples. In a medium bowl, combine remaining ¾ cup baking mix, pecans, Brown Sugar Twin, and margarine. Mix well with a fork until mixture is crumbly. Sprinkle crumb mixture evenly over top. Bake for 50 to 55 minutes or until a knife inserted in center comes out clean. Place pan on a wire rack and allow to cool for 10 to 15 minutes. Cut into 8 servings.

HINT: Good served with Cool Whip Lite, but don't forget to count the few additional calories.

Each serving equals:

HE: 1 Bread • ¾ Fruit • ¾ Fat • ¼ Skim Milk •
¼ Protein (limited) • 9 Optional Calories

178 Calories • 6 gm Fat • 5 gm Protein •
26 gm Carbohydrate • 317 mg Sodium •
97 mg Calcium • 1 gm Fiber

DIABETIC: 1 Starch/Carbohydrate • 1 Fruit • 1 Fat

Linzer-Hungarian Jam and Meringue Cake

Inspired by the remarkable Hungarian dessert, the *linzer torte*, I created my own Healthy Exchanges version that celebrates the exquisite flavors of this renowned dessert. I chose blueberry for this recipe, but you could choose to experiment with other flavors, too.

○ Serves 12

> 1 (8-serving) package Pillsbury Reduced Fat Crescent Rolls
> 1 cup blueberry spreadable fruit
> 9 egg whites
> ¾ cup Sugar Twin or Sprinkle Sweet
> 1 teaspoon coconut extract
> ¼ cup (1 ounce) chopped pecans
> 3 tablespoons flaked coconut

Preheat oven to 350 degrees. Pat crescent rolls into a rimmed 10-by-15-inch baking sheet, being sure to seal perforations. Spread spreadable fruit evenly over rolls. Bake for 12 to 15 minutes or until edges are golden brown. Place baking sheet on a wire rack while preparing meringue. Increase oven temperature to 425 degrees. In a large bowl, beat egg whites with an electric mixer on HIGH until soft peaks form. Add sugar substitute and coconut extract. Continue beating on HIGH until stiff peaks form. Spread meringue evenly over top of baked crescent rolls. Sprinkle pecans and coconut evenly over meringue. Return to oven and continue baking for 10 to 12 minutes or until meringue lightly browns. Place baking sheet on a wire rack and allow to cool. Cut into 12 servings.

HINT: Do not use inexpensive rolls, as they don't cover the pan properly.

Each serving equals:

HE: 1⅓ Fruit • ⅔ Bread • ⅓ Fat • ¼ Protein • 10 Optional Calories

153 Calories • 5 gm Fat • 3 gm Protein • 24 gm Carbohydrate • 183 mg Sodium • 2 mg Calcium • 0 gm Fiber

DIABETIC: 1 Fruit • 1 Fat • ½ Starch

Nathan's Gooey Chocolate Cake ❄

If you need an "awesome" dessert for a teenager's birthday, stir up this outrageously yummy cake I created for the graduation party of a friend's son! Does this list of ingredients—peanuts, caramel, chocolate chips—sound like "healthy" food? I'm here to show you how you can enjoy these special treats IN MODERATION.

☯ Serves 12

> 1½ cups all-purpose flour
> ¼ cup unsweetened cocoa
> 1 cup Carnation Nonfat Dry Milk Powder ☆
> 1 teaspoon baking soda
> ½ cup Sugar Twin or Sprinkle Sweet
> ¾ cup Kraft fat-free mayonnaise
> 1¾ cups water ☆
> 2½ teaspoons vanilla extract ☆
> ⅓ cup (1½ ounces) chopped dry-roasted peanuts
> 2 tablespoons (½ ounce) mini chocolate chips
> 2 tablespoons caramel syrup
> 1 (4-serving) package JELL-O sugar-free instant chocolate fudge
>   pudding mix
> ½ cup Cool Whip Free

Preheat oven to 350 degrees. Spray a 9-by-9-inch cake pan with butter-flavored cooking spray. In a large bowl, combine flour, cocoa, ⅓ cup dry milk powder, baking soda, and sugar substitute. Add mayonnaise, 1 cup water, and 1½ teaspoons vanilla extract. Mix well to combine. Pour mixture into prepared cake pan. Sprinkle peanuts and chocolate chips evenly over cake batter. Drizzle caramel syrup over the top. Using a fork, gently swirl the toppings into the cake batter. Bake for 20 to 22 minutes or until a toothpick inserted in center comes out clean. DO NOT OVERBAKE. Place cake pan on a wire rack and allow to cool completely. In a medium bowl, combine dry pudding mix, remaining ⅔ cup dry milk powder, and remaining ¾ cup water. Mix well using a wire whisk.

Blend in Cool Whip Free and remaining 1 teaspoon vanilla extract. Spread mixture evenly over cooled cake. Refrigerate for at least 30 minutes. Cut into 12 servings. Refrigerate leftovers.

Each serving equals:

HE: ⅔ Bread • ¼ Fat • ¼ Skim Milk • ½ Slider • 12 Optional Calories

151 Calories • 3 gm Fat • 5 gm Protein • 26 gm Carbohydrate • 417 mg Sodium • 79 mg Calcium • 2 gm Fiber

DIABETIC: 1½ Starch/Carbohydrate • ½ Fat

This and That

Orange Juice Spritzer

Since so many people prefer to serve non-alcoholic beverages at their parties, I'm constantly blending up new drinks that meet my requirements: easy, healthy, and yummy, too! Here's my latest way to "Dew" it, and it offers plenty of fizzy fun. ❍ Serves 6 (1 cup)

> 2 cups cold unsweetened orange juice
> 4 cups cold Diet Mountain Dew
> Orange slices (optional)

In a tall pitcher, combine orange juice and Diet Mountain Dew. Mix well. Pour over ice in 6 tall glasses. Garnish with fresh orange slices, if desired.

Each serving equals:

HE: ⅔ Fruit

32 Calories • 0 gm Fat • 0 gm Protein •
8 gm Carbohydrate • 18 mg Sodium •
7 mg Calcium • 0 gm Fiber

DIABETIC: ½ Fruit

Cape Cod Cooler

I don't care for iced tea, but Cliff sure does! I stirred this up to cool him off after he mowed our five-acre "yard" at the Healthy Exchanges Corporate Headquarters. After a glass of this, he was ready to tackle the rest of his "to-do" list with a smile!

○ Serves 4 (1 cup)

> 3 cups prepared unsweetened iced tea
> 1 cup Ocean Spray reduced-calorie cranberry juice cocktail
> Sugar substitute to equal ¼ cup sugar
> 1 teaspoon lemon juice
> Ice

In a large pitcher, combine iced tea, cranberry juice cocktail, sugar substitute, and lemon juice. Mix well to combine. For each serving, fill tall glass with ice and pour 1 cup cooler over ice.

Each serving equals:

HE: ¼ Fruit • 6 Optional Calories

20 Calories • 0 gm Fat • 0 gm Protein •
5 gm Carbohydrate • 38 mg Sodium • 0 mg Calcium •
0 gm Fiber

DIABETIC: 1 Free Food

Lite Fruit Slush

"Smoothies" are one of the hottest food trends these days, but I've been blending up great fruit combos for years, and this is one of my favorites. The frozen strawberries give this recipe lots of "oomph," so it's important not to let them thaw out.

○ Serves 12 (¾ cup)

⅔ cup (2 ripe medium) mashed bananas ☆
1 cup (one 8-ounce can) crushed pineapple, packed in fruit juice, undrained ☆
1½ cups unsweetened orange juice ☆
¼ cup Sugar Twin or Sprinkle Sweet ☆
3 cups frozen unsweetened strawberries ☆
4 cups Diet 7UP ☆

In a blender container, combine ⅓ cup banana, ½ cup undrained pineapple, ¾ cup orange juice, 2 tablespoons sugar substitute, and 1½ cups strawberries. Add 2 cups Diet 7UP. Cover and process on BLEND until mixture is smooth. Pour into a large container. Repeat with remaining fruit, orange juice, sugar substitute, and Diet 7UP. Cover and freeze. Thaw for 15 to 20 minutes before serving.

Each serving equals:

HE: 1 Fruit • 2 Optional Calories

48 Calories • 0 gm Fat • 0 gm Protein •
12 gm Carbohydrate • 10 mg Sodium •
11 mg Calcium • 1 gm Fiber

DIABETIC: 1 Fruit

Cupid's Cream

Make everyone in the family your valentine this year when you serve this frothy, refreshing treat! And when both the kids and your spouse say "Thank you," I bet it will warm the cockles of your heart. ☯ Serves 6 (1 cup)

> 2 cups Ocean Spray reduced-calorie cranberry juice cocktail
> ½ cup unsweetened orange juice
> 1 (4-serving) package JELL-O sugar-free cherry gelatin
> 3 cups Wells' Blue Bunny sugar- and fat-free vanilla ice cream

In a blender container, combine cranberry juice cocktail, orange juice, and dry gelatin. Cover and process on HIGH for 10 seconds. Add ice cream. Re-cover and continue processing on HIGH for 15 seconds or until mixture is smooth. Pour into glasses.

HINT: If you can't find Wells' Blue Bunny, use any sugar- and fat-free ice cream.

Each serving equals:

HE: ½ Fruit • ¼ Slider • 16 Optional Calories

116 Calories • 0 gm Fat • 5 gm Protein •
24 gm Carbohydrate • 98 mg Sodium •
122 mg Calcium • 0 gm Fiber

DIABETIC: 1 Fruit • 1 Starch/Carbohydrate

Chocolate Cream Soda

Bring on the hot and humid nights of summer! A refreshing cold glass of this will almost make it seem like a night under the stars in the north woods. Or, at the very least, you won't mind the heat because this tastes just that good!   ☻   Serves 4

> 2 cups skim milk
> ½ cup Nestlé Sugar-Free Chocolate Flavored Quik
> 6 to 8 ice cubes
> 1 cup club soda

In a blender container, combine skim milk and chocolate milk mix. Cover and process on BLEND for 15 seconds. Add ice cubes one at a time. Re-cover and process on PUREE for 60 seconds or until mixture is thick and ice cubes are processed. Stir in club soda. Pour evenly into 4 tall glasses.

Each serving equals:

HE: ½ Skim Milk • ½ Slider

81 Calories • 1 gm Fat • 5 gm Protein •
13 gm Carbohydrate • 120 mg Sodium •
153 mg Calcium • 2 gm Fiber

DIABETIC: ½ Skim Milk •
½ Starch/Carbohydrate *or* 1 Starch/Carbohydrate

Creamy Strawberry Fruit Dip

Both children and adults will find it fun to dip fresh fruit into this creamy dip—just wait and see! Try it with apples, with grapes, with crisp slices of pear or even firm peaches. It's an appetite-teaser and a palate-pleaser in my book.   ☻   Serves 4 (¼ cup)

¾ cup Yoplait plain fat-free yogurt
⅓ cup Carnation Nonfat Dry Milk Powder
1 teaspoon vanilla extract
Sugar substitute to equal 1 tablespoon sugar
¼ cup strawberry spreadable fruit

In a medium bowl, combine yogurt and dry milk powder. Add vanilla extract and sugar substitute. Mix well to combine. Stir in spreadable fruit. Cover and refrigerate for at least 30 minutes. Gently stir again just before serving.

Each serving equals:

HE: 1 Fruit • ½ Skim Milk • 2 Optional Calories

80 Calories • 0 gm Fat • 4 gm Protein •
16 gm Carbohydrate • 63 mg Sodium •
154 mg Calcium • 0 gm Fiber

DIABETIC: 1 Fruit •
½ Skim Milk *or* 1 Starch/Carbohydrate

Spinach and Chicken Party Dip

Here's a great choice to bring to an office party or family gathering. It's so quick to prepare, it's got something for everyone in its mélange of ingredients, and it's both creamy and crunchy! I designed this recipe to be served cold, but I also bet it would be delightful warmed up just a bit. ☻ Serves 8 (full ⅓ cup)

> 1 (8-ounce) package Philadelphia fat-free cream cheese
> ¾ cup Yoplait plain fat-free yogurt
> ⅓ cup Carnation Nonfat Dry Milk Powder
> ½ cup Kraft fat-free mayonnaise
> 2 teaspoons dried onion flakes
> 2 tablespoons dried vegetable flakes
> ¼ cup (1 ounce) chopped toasted almonds
> 1 cup (5 ounces) diced cooked chicken breast
> 1 (10-ounce) package frozen chopped spinach, thawed and
>   thoroughly drained

In a large bowl, stir cream cheese with a spoon until soft. Add yogurt, dry milk powder, and mayonnaise. Mix well to combine. Stir in onion flakes, vegetable flakes, and almonds. Add chicken and spinach. Mix well to combine. Cover and refrigerate for 1 hour. Gently stir again just before serving. Good with both vegetables and crackers.

HINTS: 1. Leftovers are wonderful on hot baked potatoes.
        2. If you don't have leftovers, purchase a chunk of cooked chicken breast from your local deli.

Each serving equals:

HE: 1¼ Protein • ¼ Fat • ¼ Skim Milk •
¼ Vegetable • 10 Optional Calories

115 Calories • 3 gm Fat • 13 gm Protein •
9 gm Carbohydrate • 373 mg Sodium •
126 mg Calcium • 1 gm Fiber

DIABETIC: 1 Meat • ½ Starch

Grande Gringo Dip

Tired of serving the same old onion dip at every festive occasion? I know I was, so I put on my sombrero one afternoon and came up with this tangy concoction that's sure to please. Cliff likes to stir in a little extra heat, but even when I tell him he looks a little funny with smoke coming from his ears, he just smiles.

● Serves 6 (½ cup)

> 1 (8-ounce) package Philadelphia fat-free cream cheese
> 1 (10¾-ounce) can Healthy Request Tomato Soup
> ¾ cup chunky salsa (mild, medium, or hot)

In a medium bowl, stir cream cheese with a spoon until soft. Add tomato soup and salsa. Mix well to combine. Cover and refrigerate for at least 30 minutes. Serve with veggies and reduced-fat crackers.

HINT: Also good on a baked potato, topped with 1 tablespoon shredded reduced-fat Cheddar cheese.

Each serving equals:

HE: ⅔ Protein • ¼ Vegetable • ¼ Slider •
10 Optional Calories

60 Calories • 0 gm Fat • 6 gm Protein •
9 gm Carbohydrate • 490 mg Sodium •
45 mg Calcium • 0 gm Fiber

DIABETIC: ½ Meat • ½ Starch/Carbohydrate

JO's Hollandaise Sauce

I was delighted to turn this traditional "No-No" into a healthy and tasty "Yes!" It took a few tries before I hit on the best combination of ingredients, but both Cliff and I were very pleased with the result. Of course, he won't eat it with broccoli, but it is also scrumptious over green beans.　　　❍　　　Serves 4 (¼ cup)

½ cup Kraft fat-free mayonnaise

½ cup Land O Lakes no-fat sour cream

2 tablespoons skim milk

2 teaspoons lemon juice

1 teaspoon prepared mustard

In a 2-cup glass measuring cup, combine mayonnaise, sour cream, and skim milk. Add lemon juice and mustard. Mix well to combine. Microwave on BRAISE (40% power) for 4 minutes, stirring after every minute.

HINT:　　Great served over cooked broccoli.

Each serving equals:

HE: ½ Slider • 13 Optional Calories

52 Calories • 0 gm Fat • 2 gm Protein •
11 gm Carbohydrate • 329 mg Sodium •
62 mg Calcium • 0 gm Fiber

DIABETIC: ½ Starch/Carbohydrate

JO's Special Sauce

No one has yet called JO's Cafe a fast-food joint, but why should we have to dine out in order to top our burgers with a very special sauce? This recipe came from lots of careful testing—not from "inside information," I promise you—but I hope you'll agree I've discovered how to prepare their big secret right at home!

○ Makes about 1½ cups (1-tablespoon serving)

1 cup Kraft fat-free mayonnaise
⅓ cup Kraft Fat-Free French Dressing
¼ cup sweet pickle relish
¼ teaspoon black pepper
1 tablespoon dried onion flakes

In a medium bowl, combine mayonnaise, French dressing, pickle relish, black pepper, and onion flakes. Mix well to combine. Cover and store in refrigerator.

Each serving equals:

HE: 16 Optional Calories

16 Calories • 0 gm Fat • 0 gm Protein •
4 gm Carbohydrate • 138 mg Sodium •
1 mg Calcium • 0 gm Fiber

DIABETIC: 1 Free Food

Shrimp Wheels

We gave these a taste-testing at one of our monthly Healthy Exchanges birthday parties, and everyone agreed they tasted as yummy as they looked! I think they'd be ideal for a holiday party, since they bake up a dozen at a time and so easily. Go ahead, celebrate—it's good for you! ☻ Serves 12 (2 each)

2 tablespoons Kraft fat-free mayonnaise
2 tablespoons chili sauce
1 tablespoon finely chopped celery
1 (4.5-ounce drained weight) can small shrimp, rinsed and
    drained
1 (8-ounce) can Pillsbury Reduced Fat Crescent Rolls

Preheat oven to 375 degrees. In a medium bowl, combine mayonnaise, chili sauce, celery, and shrimp. Mix well to combine. Unroll dough and separate into 4 rectangles. Spread about ¼ cup shrimp mixture over each section of dough. Roll up each section and refrigerate for 15 minutes. Cut each into 6 slices. Arrange slices on ungreased baking sheet. Bake for 10 to 12 minutes or until browned. Serve hot. Leftovers reheat well in microwave.

HINT: Tuna or crab meat may be substituted for shrimp.

Each serving equals:

HE: ⅔ Bread • ⅓ Protein • 6 Optional Calories

79 Calories • 3 gm Fat • 4 gm Protein •
9 gm Carbohydrate • 196 mg Sodium •
7 mg Calcium • 0 gm Fiber

DIABETIC: ½ Starch • ½ Fat

Bavarian Party Rye Treats

Remember that old sixties tune, "It's My Party"? Well, this time it's *your* party, so instead of crying, you can smile as you offer your guests a platter of this cocktail–party pleaser! It makes a terrific go-along if you're planning an Oktoberfest beer-tasting party or just a postgame buffet. ● Serves 8 (3 each)

¼ cup Kraft fat-free mayonnaise

½ cup Land O Lakes no-fat sour cream

2 teaspoons Brown Sugar Twin

1 teaspoon caraway seeds

2 teaspoons dried parsley flakes

1 teaspoon dried onion flakes

1 cup (one 8-ounce can) sauerkraut, well drained

2 (¾-ounce) slices Kraft reduced-fat Swiss cheese, shredded

½ cup (3 ounces) finely diced Dubuque 97% fat-free ham or any
    extra-lean ham

24 pumpernickel bread rounds or squares

In a large bowl, combine mayonnaise, sour cream, Brown Sugar Twin, caraway seeds, parsley flakes, and onion flakes. Add sauerkraut, Swiss cheese, and ham. Mix well to combine. Spoon about 1 tablespoon mixture over each bread round. Cover and refrigerate for at least 30 minutes.

Each serving equals:

HE: 1 Bread • ½ Protein • ¼ Vegetable • ¼ Slider •
2 Optional Calories

---

131 Calories • 3 gm Fat • 6 gm Protein •
20 gm Carbohydrate • 627 mg Sodium •
50 mg Calcium • 3 gm Fiber

DIABETIC: 1 Starch • 1 Meat

Cheese-Dill Tarts

These "mini-quiches" are another great party snack. They taste so good, your guests may not believe that what they're enjoying is also good for them. Just smile and say, "Believe what you will!" Couldn't you survive a lifetime of living this well? I could!

♥ Serves 8 (two each)

> 1 Pillsbury refrigerated unbaked 9-inch piecrust
> 1⅓ cups Carnation Nonfat Dry Milk Powder
> ½ cup water
> 1 egg, beaten, or equivalent in egg substitute
> ¼ cup (¾ ounce) grated Kraft fat-free Parmesan cheese
> ½ teaspoon dill weed
> ⅛ teaspoon black pepper
> ⅓ cup (1½ ounces) shredded Kraft reduced-fat Cheddar cheese

Preheat oven to 400 degrees. Unfold piecrust. Using a 2½-inch biscuit cutter, cut 12 circles. Press dough scraps together and cut out 4 more circles, for a total of 16 circles. Place pastry circles into 16 miniature muffin cups. Press to form tarts. In a large bowl, combine dry milk powder and water. Stir in egg, Parmesan cheese, dill weed, and black pepper. Add Cheddar cheese. Mix well to combine. Evenly spoon mixture into pastry shells. Bake for 18 to 22 minutes or until light brown. Serve hot or cold.

Each serving equals:

HE: ½ Protein • ½ Bread • ½ Skim Milk •
½ Slider • 10 Optional Calories

193 Calories • 9 gm Fat • 7 gm Protein •
21 gm Carbohydrate • 269 mg Sodium •
177 mg Calcium • 0 gm Fiber

DIABETIC: 1 Starch • 1 Fat • ½ Meat •
½ Skim Milk

Breakfast Biscuits

Fresh biscuits in the morning in about 15 minutes? Does it seem like an impossibility? Well, the proof is in the eating, and you'll see some speedy gobbling by all members of the family when these emerge from the oven, fragrant and sweet.   ☻   Serves 8

> 1½ cups Bisquick Reduced Fat Baking Mix
> ¼ cup + 1 tablespoon Sugar Twin or Sprinkle Sweet ☆
> ½ cup raisins
> ¼ cup Kraft fat-free mayonnaise
> ¾ cup water
> ½ teaspoon ground cinnamon

Preheat oven to 415 degrees. Spray 8 wells of a 12-hole muffin pan with butter-flavored cooking spray, or line with paper liners. In a medium bowl, combine baking mix, ¼ cup sugar substitute, and raisins. Add mayonnaise and water. Mix well to combine. Fill prepared muffin wells half full. In a small bowl, combine cinnamon and remaining 1 tablespoon Sugar Twin. Sprinkle cinnamon mixture evenly over biscuits. Cut mixture into biscuits with a knife. Bake for 10 to 12 minutes. Place muffin pan on a wire rack and let set for 5 minutes. Serve warm.

HINT: Fill unused muffin wells with water. It protects the muffin tin and ensures even baking.

Each serving equals:

HE: 1 Bread • ½ Fruit • 9 Optional Calories

113 Calories • 1 gm Fat • 2 gm Protein •
24 gm Carbohydrate • 327 mg Sodium •
24 mg Calcium • 1 gm Fiber

DIABETIC: 1 Starch • ½ Fruit

Easy Sticky Buns

If you've got five extra minutes to spare, you can throw these quick breakfast treats into the oven and go about your business of getting ready for the day. Come back 15 minutes later and enjoy! Take it from me—don't leave home without filling your tummy with satisfying food. It really is easier to stick to a sound eating plan for the rest of the day. ❍ Serves 5 (2 each)

> ⅓ cup Cary's Sugar Free Maple Syrup
> ½ cup + 2 tablespoons raisins
> 1 (7.5-ounce) can Pillsbury refrigerated biscuits

Preheat oven to 350 degrees. Pour maple syrup into a 9-inch pie plate. Add raisins. Mix well to combine. Divide dough into 10 biscuits and arrange on top of maple syrup mixture. Lightly spray top of biscuits with butter-flavored cooking spray. Bake for 15 minutes or until golden brown. Invert onto serving plate and serve warm.

Each serving equals:

HE: 1½ Bread • 1 Fruit • 11 Optional Calories

169 Calories • 1 gm Fat • 3 gm Protein •
37 gm Carbohydrate • 402 mg Sodium •
9 mg Calcium • 3 gm Fiber

DIABETIC: 1½ Starch • 1 Fruit

Maple Cornbread Muffins ❄

This unusual mix of flavors should make your taste buds stand up and cheer! The sweet and crunchy ingredients join hands beautifully with classic cornbread, and the result offers a fresh take on a traditional recipe. ☻ Serves 8

> 1 cup (6 ounces) yellow cornmeal
> 6 tablespoons all-purpose flour
> ¼ cup Sugar Twin or Sprinkle Sweet
> 1 teaspoon baking powder
> ½ teaspoon baking soda
> ¼ cup (1 ounce) chopped walnuts
> ⅔ cup Carnation Nonfat Dry Milk Powder
> ½ cup water
> 1 egg or equivalent in egg substitute
> ½ cup Cary's Sugar Free Maple Syrup

Preheat oven to 425 degrees. Spray 8 wells of a 12-hole muffin pan with butter-flavored cooking spray, or line with paper liners. In a large bowl, combine cornmeal, flour, sugar substitute, baking powder, baking soda, and walnuts. In a small bowl, combine dry milk powder and water. Add egg and maple syrup. Mix well to combine. Stir milk mixture into cornmeal mixture. Spoon batter evenly into prepared muffin wells. Bake for 10 to 14 minutes or until a toothpick inserted in center comes out clean. Place muffin pan on a wire rack and let set for 5 minutes. Remove muffins from pan and continue cooling on wire rack.

HINT: Fill unused muffin wells with water. It protects the muffin tin and ensures even baking.

Each serving equals:

HE: 1¼ Bread • ¼ Fat • ¼ Protein • ¼ Skim Milk •
13 Optional Calories

143 Calories • 3 gm Fat • 5 gm Protein •
24 gm Carbohydrate • 213 mg Sodium •
111 mg Calcium • 2 gm Fiber

DIABETIC: 1½ Starch • ½ Fat

Carrot-Banana Bread

Instead of a standard banana bread, why not delight your family with this crunchy-sweet version that delivers extra-good nutrition (especially vitamin A in those carrots)? As for whether I prefer 8 thick or 16 thin slices, it really depends on the day. Sometimes I like the cozy old-fashioned feeling a substantial slice delivers; other days, I find I feel more satisfied by enjoying two slices instead of just one.   ☻   Serves 8 (1 thick or 2 thin slices)

> 1½ cups all-purpose flour
> 1 (4-serving) package JELL-O sugar-free instant vanilla pudding mix
> 2 tablespoons Brown Sugar Twin
> 1 teaspoon baking soda
> ½ teaspoon baking powder
> 1 teaspoon ground cinnamon
> ¼ cup (1 ounce) chopped walnuts
> 1 cup grated carrots
> ⅔ cup (2 ripe medium) mashed bananas
> ¾ cup unsweetened applesauce
> 1 egg or equivalent in egg substitute

Preheat oven to 350 degrees. Spray a 9-by-5-inch loaf pan with butter-flavored cooking spray. In a large bowl, combine flour, dry pudding mix, Brown Sugar Twin, baking soda, baking powder, and cinnamon. Stir in walnuts and carrots. In a small bowl, combine bananas, applesauce, and egg. Add banana mixture to flour mixture. Mix gently just to combine. Spread batter into prepared loaf pan. Bake for 50 to 60 minutes or until a toothpick inserted in center comes out clean. Place pan on a wire rack and allow to cool for 5 minutes. Remove from pan and continue cooling on wire rack. Cut into 8 thick or 16 thin slices.

Each serving equals:

HE: 1 Bread • ⅔ Fruit • ¼ Protein • ¼ Fat •
¼ Vegetable • 14 Optional Calories

155 Calories • 3 gm Fat • 4 gm Protein •
28 gm Carbohydrate • 259 mg Sodium •
35 mg Calcium • 2 gm Fiber

DIABETIC: 1 Starch • 1 Fruit • ½ Fat

Apricot Oatmeal Bread

Quick tea breads are a healthy baker's secret weapon because they're easy to stir up, they freeze beautifully, and they just brim with that homemade look and taste. The dried apricots are a surprising but truly delightful treat, and the oats give it a wonderfully hearty texture.   ☺   Serves 8 (1 thick or 2 thin slices)

1½ cups Bisquick Reduced-Fat Baking Mix
¾ cup (2¼ ounces) quick oats
⅔ cup Carnation Nonfat Dry Milk Powder
1 teaspoon baking powder
3 tablespoons Sugar Twin or Sprinkle Sweet
¾ cup (3 ounces) chopped dried apricots
¼ cup (1 ounce) chopped walnuts
1¼ cups water
1 egg, beaten, or equivalent in egg substitute

Preheat oven to 350 degrees. Spray a 9-by-5-inch loaf pan with butter-flavored cooking spray. In a large bowl, combine baking mix, oats, dry milk powder, baking powder, sugar substitute, apricots, and walnuts. Add water and egg. Blend only to mix. Pour batter into prepared loaf pan. Bake for 40 to 45 minutes or until a toothpick inserted near center comes out clean. Place pan on a wire rack and let set for 5 minutes. Remove from pan and continue cooling on wire rack. Cut into 8 thick or 16 thin slices.

Each serving equals:

HE: 1½ Bread • ½ Fruit • ¼ Fat • ¼ Skim Milk •
¼ Protein • 2 Optional Calories

197 Calories • 5 gm Fat • 6 gm Protein •
32 gm Carbohydrate • 363 mg Sodium •
137 mg Calcium • 2 gm Fiber

DIABETIC: 1½ Starch • ½ Fruit •
½ Fat *or* 2 Starch/Carbohydrate • ½ Fat

Iowa Homestead Pancakes ❄

I like trying to make the everyday meal a little extra-special because I think you're worth it! Here's the kind of recipe you might expect to be served at a ritzy country inn, but it belongs just as well at your kitchen table. And no, I don't put corn in *everything* I stir up. I'm just a proud Iowan! ◐ Serves 6

1½ cups Bisquick Reduced-Fat Baking Mix
⅔ cup Carnation Nonfat Dry Milk Powder
½ cup frozen whole-kernel corn, thawed
1 full cup (6 ounces) finely diced Dubuque 97% fat-free ham or any extra-lean ham
1 cup water
¾ cup Cary's Sugar Free Maple Syrup

In a medium bowl, combine baking mix and dry milk powder. Stir in corn and ham. Add water. Mix well to combine. Using a ⅓ cup measure as a guide, spread batter onto a griddle or in a large skillet sprayed with butter-flavored cooking spray to form 6 pancakes. Flatten slightly with spatula. Cook over medium heat until pancakes are browned on both sides. For each serving, place 1 pancake on a plate and pour 2 tablespoons warm syrup over top.

HINTS: 1. Thaw corn by placing in a colander and rinsing under hot water for one minute.
2. Warm syrup in microwave while preparing pancakes.

Each serving equals:

HE: 1½ Bread • ⅔ Protein • ⅓ Skim Milk • ¼ Slider

199 Calories • 3 gm Fat • 10 gm Protein •
33 gm Carbohydrate • 698 mg Sodium •
116 mg Calcium • 1 gm Fiber

DIABETIC: 2 Starch • 1 Meat

Aloha Pancakes

These are almost like having dessert for breakfast—and they're a true favorite of my grandson Zach, the boy we fondly call "the Pancake Kid." What a great way to celebrate the start of a brand-new day, and what a loving way to show your family how much you care. ☻ Serves 6 (2 each)

> 1½ cups Aunt Jemima Reduced Calorie Pancake Mix
> 2 tablespoons (½ ounce) chopped pecans
> 1 cup (one 8-ounce can) crushed pineapple, packed in fruit juice,
>   undrained
> ½ cup Cary's Sugar Free Maple Syrup
> ⅔ cup water

In a large bowl, combine pancake mix and pecans. In a medium bowl, combine undrained pineapple, maple syrup, and water. Add pineapple mixture to pancake mixture. Mix gently with a wire whisk just until blended. Using a ¼ cup measure as a guide, pour batter onto a large griddle or into a skillet sprayed with butter-flavored cooking spray. Gently spread with rubber spatula or spoon to form 12 (4-inch) round pancakes. Cook over medium heat until pancakes are browned on both sides.

HINT: Serve with additional maple syrup or apple butter.

Each serving equals:

HE: 1⅓ Bread • ⅓ Fat • ⅓ Fruit •
13 Optional Calories

---

170 Calories • 2 gm Fat • 6 gm Protein •
32 gm Carbohydrate • 432 mg Sodium •
189 mg Calcium • 4 gm Fiber

DIABETIC: 2 Starch/Carbohydrate

New England Ham Omelet

One morning when it was just the two of us, I decided to make a ham omelet for Sunday breakfast. Then I spotted an onion and an apple, and inspiration struck! The maple syrup may seem an odd choice for eggs, but it gives the ham a little extra pizazz!

❂ Serves 2

1/4 cup chopped onion
1/2 cup (1 small) cored, unpeeled, and diced cooking apple
1/4 cup (1 1/2 ounces) diced Dubuque 97% fat-free ham or any
 extra-lean ham
2 tablespoons Cary's Sugar Free Maple Syrup
3 eggs or equivalent in egg substitute
1/4 teaspoon lemon pepper

In a medium skillet sprayed with butter-flavored cooking spray, sauté onion, apple, and ham for 5 minutes or until browned. Add maple syrup. Mix well to combine. Lower heat and simmer while preparing eggs. In a medium bowl, combine eggs and lemon pepper. Beat well with a fork. Spray a large skillet with butter-flavored cooking spray. Pour egg mixture into skillet. Cook over high heat for 1 minute. Lower heat. Stir eggs rapidly with a wooden spoon. Gently pat egg mixture back into place and continue cooking without stirring, 1 minute. Add ham filling to bottom half. Flip top half over. Cut in half and serve at once.

Each serving equals:

HE: 2 Protein (1 1/2 limited) • 1/2 Fruit • 1/4 Vegetable • 10 Optional Calories

160 Calories • 8 gm Fat • 13 gm Protein • 9 gm Carbohydrate • 309 mg Sodium • 43 mg Calcium • 1 gm Fiber

DIABETIC: 2 Meat • 1/2 Fruit

Italian Baked Zucchini Omelet

If you've always made your omelet in a skillet, I'd like you to try something fresh and new. This flavorful dish bakes up beautifully in your oven and looks truly luscious when you serve it. It's a great way to get those good-for-you veggies at breakfast or brunch, as well as lots of healthy protein.   ♥   Serves 4

> ¼ cup Kraft Fat-Free Italian Dressing
> ½ cup chopped onion
> 2 cups shredded unpeeled zucchini
> 4 eggs, beaten, or equivalent in egg substitute
> ¼ cup (¾ ounce) grated Kraft fat-free Parmesan cheese
> ¼ teaspoon lemon pepper

Preheat oven to 400 degrees. Spray an 8-by-8-inch baking dish with butter-flavored cooking spray. In a large skillet, heat Italian dressing. Add onion and zucchini. Cook over medium heat for 4 to 5 minutes or until zucchini is slightly wilted, stirring often. Remove from heat. Cool for 2 to 3 minutes. In a large bowl, combine eggs, Parmesan cheese, and lemon pepper. Mix well with a wire whisk until fluffy. Stir in zucchini mixture. Pour egg mixture into prepared baking dish. Bake for 22 to 26 minutes or until firm. Place baking dish on a wire rack and let set for 5 minutes. Divide into 4 servings.

Each serving equals:

> HE: 1¼ Vegetable • 1¼ Protein (1 limited) •
> 8 Optional Calories
>
> ---
>
> 117 Calories • 5 gm Fat • 8 gm Protein •
> 10 gm Carbohydrate • 333 mg Sodium •
> 38 mg Calcium • 2 gm Fiber
>
> ---
>
> DIABETIC: 1½ Meat • 1 Vegetable

Heart Smart Menus for the Entire Family

"Let's Fall in Love" Valentine's Day Dinner

Valentine Party Salad
Mushroom-Scalloped Potatoes
Chicken Breast with Corn-Walnut Salsa
Barbara's Heavenly Chocolate Pie
Cupid's Cream

March Madness Sports Supper

Heartland Corn Chowder
Sweet Potato Salad
Deviled Green Beans
Momma's Porcupine Meatballs
Mexican Pot Pie
Partyline Kahlua Cheesecake

Let's Celebrate Spring Luncheon

Inn of the Six-Toed Cat Pea Salad
Denise's Spring Dew Salad
Creamed Chicken with Cornbread Shortcakes
Riviera Strawberry Pie
Orange Juice Spritzer

Family Fourth of July Potluck

Dad's Potato Salad
Carrot Picnic Salad
Barbecue Burgers
Iowa Farm Boy Reubens
Fresh Peach-Blueberry Pie
Cape Cod Cooler

Hearty Harvest Buffet

James's Quick and Thick Chili
Harvest Chicken Skillet
Creamy Broccoli and Ham Bake
He-Man Baked Beans
Chocolate-Covered Cherry Cordial Pie
Winter Strawberry-Rhubarb Cobbler

Deck the Halls Holiday Party

Bavarian Party Rye Treats
Spinach and Chicken Party Dip
Mountain Cranberry Holiday Salad
Chicken Apple Swiss Bake
Sauerbraten Meatballs
Crock Pot Party Beans
Chocolate Pecan Layered Pie
Oatmeal Chocolate Chip Cookies

Making Healthy Exchanges Work for You

You're ready now to begin a wonderful journey to better health. In the preceding pages, you've discovered the remarkable variety of good food available to you when you begin eating the Healthy Exchanges way. You've stocked your pantry and learned many of my food preparation "secrets" that will point you on the way to delicious success.

But before I let you go, I'd like to share a few tips that I've learned while traveling toward healthier eating habits. It took me a long time to learn how to eat *smarter*. In fact, I'm still working on it. But I am getting better. For years, I could *inhale* a five-course meal in five minutes flat—and still make room for a second helping of dessert!

Now I follow certain signposts on the road that help me stay on the right path. I hope these ideas will help point you in the right direction as well.

1. **Eat slowly** so your brain has time to catch up with your tummy. Cut and chew each bite slowly. Try putting your fork down between bites. Stop eating as soon as you feel full. Crumple your napkin and throw it on top of your plate so you don't continue to eat when you are no longer hungry.

2. **Smaller plates** may help you feel more satisfied by your food portions *and* limit the amount you can put on the plate.

3. **Watch portion size.** If you are *truly* hungry, you can always add more food to your plate once you've finished your initial serving. But remember to count the additional food accordingly.

4. **Always eat at your dining-room or kitchen table.** You deserve better than nibbling from an open refrigerator or over the sink. Make an attractive place setting, even if you're eating alone. Feed your eyes as well as your stomach. By always eating at a table, you will become much more aware of your true food intake. For some reason, many of us conveniently "forget" the food we swallow while standing over the stove or munching in the car or on the run.

5. **Avoid doing anything else while you are eating.** If you read the paper or watch television while you eat, it's easy to consume too much food without realizing it, because you are concentrating on something else besides what you're eating. Then, when you look down at your plate and see that it's empty, you wonder where all the food went and why you still feel hungry.

Day by day, as you travel the path to good health, it will become easier to make the right choices, to eat *smarter*. But don't ever fool yourself into thinking that you'll be able to put your eating habits on cruise control and forget about them. Making a commitment to eat good healthy food and sticking to it takes some effort. But with all the good-tasting recipes in this Healthy Exchanges cookbook, just think how well you're going to eat—and enjoy it—from now on!

Healthy Lean Bon Appétit!

Index

281

I want to hear from you . . .

Besides my family, the love of my life is creating "common folk" healthy recipes and solving everyday cooking questions in the *Healthy Exchanges Way*. Everyone who uses my recipes is considered part of the Healthy Exchanges Family, so please write to me if you have any questions, comments, or suggestions. I will do my best to answer. With your support, I'll continue to stir up even more recipes and cooking tips for the Family in the years to come.

Write to: JoAnna M. Lund
c/o Healthy Exchanges, Inc.
P.O. Box 124
DeWitt, IA 52742

If you prefer, you can fax me at 1-319-659-2126 or contact me via e-mail by writing to HealthyJo@aol.com. Or visit my Healthy Exchanges Internet web site at: http://www.healthyexchanges.com

Healthy Exchanges recipes are a great way to begin—
but if your goal is living healthy for a lifetime,

You Need HELP!

JoAnna M. Lund's
Healthy Exchanges Lifetime Plan

"I lost 130 pounds and reclaimed my health by following a Four Part
Plan that emphasizes not only Healthy Eating, but also Moderate
Exercise, Lifestyle Changes and Goal-Setting, and most important of
all, Positive Attitude."

- If you've lost weight before but failed to keep it off . . .
- If you've got diabetes, high blood pressure, high cholesterol, or
  heart disease—and you need to reinvent your lifestyle . . .
- If you want to raise a healthy family and encourage good lifelong
  habits in your kids . . .

HELP is on the way!

- The Support You Need • The Motivation You Want •
  A Program That Works•

HELP: Healthy Exchanges Lifetime Plan is available
at your favorite bookstore.

About the Author

JoAnna M. Lund, a graduate of the University of Western Illinois, worked as a commercial insurance underwriter for eighteen years before starting her own business, Healthy Exchanges, Inc., which publishes cookbooks, a monthly newsletter, motivational booklets, and inspirational audiotapes. Her first book, *Healthy Exchanges Cookbook*, has more than 500,000 copies in print. A popular speaker with hospitals, support groups for heart patients and diabetics, and service and volunteer organizations, she appears regularly on QVC and on regional television and radio shows, and has been featured in newspapers and magazines across the country.

The recipient of numerous business awards, JoAnna was an Iowa delegate to the national White House Conference on Small Business. She is a member of the International Association of Culinary Professionals, the Society for Nutrition Education, and other professional publishing and marketing associations. She lives with her husband, Clifford, in DeWitt, Iowa.

Susan M. Fitzgerald, R.N., M.S., is a Clinical Practice Specialist at the Inova Heart Center at Fairfax Hospital in northern Virginia, where she works continually to improve the care provided to cardiac patients. Her practice has focused on cardiology for more than fifteen years, and she has lectured both locally and at national conferences on a variety of cardiac issues. She lives in Maryland with her husband and three children.

Now That You've Seen
The Heart Smart Healthy Exchanges Cookbook, Why Not Order *The Healthy Exchanges Food Newsletter?*

If you enjoyed the recipes in this cookbook and would like to cook up even more of these "common folk" healthy dishes, you may want to subsribe to *The Healthy Exchanges Food Newsletter*.

This monthly 12-page newsletter contains 30-plus new recipes *every month,* in such columns as:

- Reader Exchange
- Reader Requests
- Recipe Makeover
- Micro Corner
- Dinner for Two

- Crock-Pot Luck
- Meatless Main Dishes
- Rise & Shine
- Our Small World

- Brown Bagging It
- Snack Attack
- Side Dishes
- Main Dishes
- Desserts

In addition to all the recipes, other regular features include:

- The Editor's Motivational Corner
- Dining Out Question & Answer
- Cooking Question & Answer
- New Product Alert
- Success Profiles of Winners in the Losing Game
- Exercise Advice from a Cardiac Rehab Specialist
- Nutrition Advice from a Registered Dietitian
- Positive Thought for the Month

Just as in this cookbook, all *Healthy Exchanges Food Newsletter* recipes are calculated in three distinct ways: 1) Weight Loss Choices, 2) Calories with Fat and Fiber Grams, and 3) Diabetic Exchanges.

The cost for a one-year (12-issue) subscription with a special Healthy Exchanges 3-ring binder to store the newsletters in is $28.50, or $22.50 without the binder. To order, simply complete the form and mail to us *or* call our toll-free number and pay with your VISA or MasterCard.

_____ Yes, I want to subscribe to *The Healthy Exchanges Food Newsletter.* $28.50 Yearly Subscription Cost with Storage Binder $_____

$22.50 Yearly Subscription Cost without Binder . . . . $_____

_____ Foreign orders please add $6.00 for money exchange and extra postage. . . . . $_____

_____ I'm not sure, so please send me a sample copy at $2.50 . . . . $_____

Please make check payable to HEALTHY EXCHANGES or pay by VISA/MasterCard

CARD NUMBER: _____ EXPIRATION DATE: _____

SIGNATURE: _____

Signature required for all credit card orders.

Or Order Toll-Free, using your credit card, at 1-800-766-8961

NAME:_____

ADDRESS:_____

CITY: _____ STATE: _____ ZIP: _____

TELEPHONE: (   ) _____

If additional orders for the newsletter are to be sent to an address other than the one listed above, please use a separate sheet and attach to this form.

MAIL TO: **HEALTHY EXCHANGES**
P.O. BOX 124
DeWitt, IA 52742-0124

1-800-766-8961 for customer orders
1-319-659-8234 for customer service

Thank you for your order, and for choosing to become a part of the Healthy Exchanges Family!

Other delicious titles by JoAnna Lund available from Putnam:

Dessert Every Night!
ISBN 0-399-14422-6 • $21.95 ($30.00 CAN)

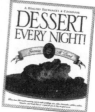

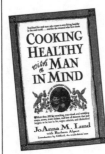

Cooking Healthy with a Man in Mind
ISBN 0-399-14265-7
$19.95 ($27.99 CAN)

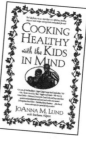

Cooking Healthy with the Kids in Mind
ISBN 0-399-14358-0 • $19.95 ($26.95 CAN)

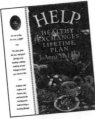

HELP: Healthy Exchanges® Lifetime Plan
ISBN 0-399-14164-2
$21.95 ($30.99 CAN)

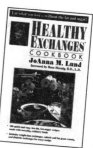

Healthy Exchanges® Cookbook
ISBN 0-399-14065-4 • $16.95 ($23.99 CAN)

Available wherever books are sold